Lange Instant Access:
Hospital Admissions

**Essential Evidence-Based Orders
for Common Clinical Conditions**

T0198122

Anil Patel, MD

Family Medicine, Class of 2006
University of Pittsburgh Medical Center (UPMC)
Pittsburgh, Pennsylvania

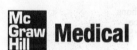

Medical

New York   Chicago   San Francisco   Lisbon   London
Madrid   Mexico City   Milan   New Delhi   San Juan   Seoul
Singapore   Sydney   Toronto

The McGraw·Hill Companies

Lange Instant Access:
Hospital Admissions: Essential Evidence-Based Orders for Common
Clinical Conditions

21 22 23 CD CD 26 25 24 23

ISBN-13: 978-0-07-148137-3
ISBN-10: 0-07-148137-0

Notice

Medicine is an ever-changing science. As new research and clinical
experience broaden our knowledge, changes in treatment and drug
therapy are required. The authors and the publisher of this work have
checked with sources believed to be reliable in their efforts to provide
information that is complete and generally in accord with the standards
accepted at the time of publication. However, in view of the possibility
of human error or changes in medical sciences, neither the authors nor
the publisher nor any other party who has been involved in the
preparation or publication of this work warrants that the information
contained herein is in every respect accurate or complete, and they
disclaim all responsibility for any errors or omissions or for the results
obtained from use of the information contained in this work. Readers are
encouraged to confirm the information contained herein with other
sources. For example, and in particular, readers are advised to check the
product information sheet included in the package of each drug they
plan to administer to be certain that the information contained in this
work is accurate and that changes have not been made in the
recommended dose or in the contraindications for administration. This
recommendation is of particular importance in connection with new or
infrequently used drugs.

This book was set in Times New Roman by Silverchair Science +
    Communications, Inc.
The editors were Jim Shanahan and Maya Barahona.
The production supervisor was Sherri Souffrance.
Project management was performed by Silverchair Science + Communications, Inc.
RR Donnelley was the printer and binder.

This book is printed on acid-free paper.

Cataloging-in-Publication data for this title is on file with the
Library of Congress.

Contents

Contents

Contributing Editors

Sheila Alas, MD
Chief Resident, Family Medicine
UPMC, Pittsburgh, Pennsylvania

Robert Barnabei, MD
Inpatient Director & Clinical Instructor, Family Medicine
UPMC, Pittsburgh, Pennsylvania

David Garzarelli, MD
Associate Program Director & Clinical Assistant Professor
Family Medicine
UPMC, Pittsburgh, Pennsylvania

Vijay Karajala, MD
Chief Resident, Internal Medicine
UPMC, Pittsburgh, Pennsylvania

Stasia Miaskiewicz, MD
Program Director, Internal Medicine
UPMC, Pittsburgh, Pennsylvania

Gustavo Ortiz, MD
Resident, PGY IV, Neurology
Jackson Memorial Hospital, University of Miami, Miami, Florida

Thomas Powell, MD
Clinical Instructor, Nephrology
UPMC, Pittsburgh, Pennsylvania

Joseph Secosky, MD
Clinical Instructor, Cardiology
UPMC, Pittsburgh, Pennsylvania

Shripal Shrishrimal, MD
Critical Care Fellow
UPMC, Pittsburgh, Pennsylvania

Phoebe Tobiano, MD
Family Medicine, Class of 2006
UPMC, Pittsburgh, Pennsylvania

Walton C. Toy, MD
Rheumatology Fellow
University of Arkansas Medical Sciences, Little Rock, Arkansas

Preface

Writing hospital admissions orders is an important and fundamental responsibility of the hospital-based physician. Surprisingly, there are few resources available to help interns and residents write the most focused and medically necessary admitting orders possible.

Lange Instant Access: Hospital Admissions: Essential Evidence-Based Orders for Common Clinical Conditions focuses on medical conditions that hospital-based physicians commonly encounter.

From cardiology to toxicology, admitting orders for dozens of diseases and disorders are presented in handy, easy-access tables. The content of each table provides the reader with a snapshot of the most important considerations for initial admissions as well as for immediate follow-up and patient management.

Lange Instant Access: Hospital Admissions includes evidence-based information, essential for today's learning and practice. All the information in the manual was acquired from respected references in the medical literature, and the appropriate citations are included throughout the manual.

This manual is a final product of 3 years of hard work, which was reviewed by some of the most recognized and respected physicians in internal medicine, family medicine, and medicine subspecialties.

Here is what some of my colleagues have to say about the manual:

- "The one and only complete and concise manual for commonly encountered admissions."

- "This is an excellent evidence-based book that eliminates carrying multiple books by having information at your fingertips like disposition of the patient, diagnostic studies, activity level of the patient, what to avoid, and finally the management of the patient's condition."

- "A good evidence-based admission reference guide for the interns and residents."

- "Useful for inpatient care as a thorough index when doing admissions and reviewing differential diagnosis."

Acknowledgments

I would like to dedicate *Lange Instant Access: Hospital Admissions* to my grandmother who had a lot of influence in my becoming a physician.

I would like to thank all the editors and contributors for their time and hard work devoted to this book. Without their efforts, this manual would not be possible. I would especially like to thank my sweetheart for her support. I also would like to thank Nina Tomaino, James Shanahan, Maya Barahona, and Melissa Jones and her team for working very closely with me in making *Lange Instant Access: Hospital Admissions* a reality.

Guide Tables

TABLE GT–1: Abbreviations	
?	Clinical correlation required
AAA	Abdominal aortic aneurysm
ABCs	Airway, breathing, circulation
ABG	Arterial blood gases
ac	Before meals
ACE	Angiotensin-converting enzyme
ACV	Assist-control ventilation
ADH	Antidiuretic hormone
AFB	Acid-fast bacilli
AIN	Acute interstitial nephritis
ALT	Alanine aminotransferase
ANA	Antinuclear antibodies
ANCA	Antineutrophil cytoplasmic antibodies
ARB	Angiotensin receptor blockers
ASA	Acetylsalicylic acid (aspirin)
5-ASA	5-Aminosalicylic acid
AST	Aspartate aminotransferase
AV	Atrioventricular
AVM	Arteriovenous malformation
BGM	Blood glucose monitor
β-HCG	β-Human chorionic gonadotropin
BMP	Basic metabolic profile (Na^+, K^+, CO_2, Cl, BUN, Cr, glucose)
BNP	B-type natriuretic peptide
BP	Blood pressure
BPH	Benign prostatic hyperplasia
BRP	Bathroom privileges
CBC	Complete blood count

(continued)

TABLE GT–1: Abbreviations (Continued)	
CHF	Congestive heart failure
CI	Cardiac index
CMP	Complete metabolic profile (BMP + LFT)
CMV	Cytomegalovirus
CNS	Central nervous system
CO	Cardiac output
COPD	Chronic obstructive pulmonary disease
CPK	Creatine phosphokinase
CRP	C-reactive protein
C&S	Culture and sensitivity
CT	Computed tomography
CVA	Cerebrovascular accident
Cx	Culture
CXR	Chest x-ray
DBP	Diastolic blood pressure
DIC	Disseminated intravascular coagulation
DM	Diabetes mellitus
DNR	Do not resuscitate
DVT	Deep vein thrombosis
Dx studies	Diagnostic studies
EBV	Epstein-Barr virus
ECG	Electrocardiogram
EEG	Electroencephalogram
EF	Ejection fraction
EGD	Esophagogastroduodenoscopy
ESR	Erythrocyte sedimentation rate
ETOH	Alcohol

(continued)

TABLE GT–1: Abbreviations (Continued)	
FFP	Fresh frozen plasma
FHx	Family history
GBM	Glomerular basement membrane
GC	Gonorrhea
GERD	Gastroesophageal reflux disease
GFR	Glomerular filtration rate
GI	Gastrointestinal
GU	Genitourinary
H&H	Hemoglobin and hematocrit
HIDA	Hepatobiliary iminodiacetic acid
HIV	Human immunodeficiency virus
HSV	Herpes simplex virus
HTN	Hypertension
IBD	Inflammatory bowel disease
ID	Infectious disease
IHSS	Idiopathic hypertrophic subaortic stenosis
INR	International normalized ratio
I/O	Intake and output
JVD	Jugular venous distention
KOH	Potassium hydroxide
KUB	Kidney, ureter, bladder
LAD	Left anterior descending
LDH	Lactate dehydrogenase
LFT	Liver function test (AST, ALT, Alk PO_4, albumin, bilirubin)
LP	Lumbar puncture
LR	Lactated Ringer's

(continued)

TABLE GT–1: Abbreviations (Continued)	
MAT	Multifocal atrial tachycardia
MDI	Metered-dose inhaler
MI	Myocardial infarction
MIVF	Maintenance IV fluid
MRI	Magnetic resonance imaging
NC	Nasal cannula
NCV	Nerve conduction velocity
NPO	Nothing by mouth
NR	No response
NS	Normal saline
N/V	Nausea/vomiting
OOB	Out of bed
p-ANCA	Perinuclear antineutrophil cytoplasmic antibodies
PCI	Percutaneous coronary intervention
PCN	Penicillin
PE	Pulmonary embolism
PET	Positron emission tomography
PFT	Pulmonary function testing
PID	Pelvic inflammatory disease
PPD	Purified protein derivative
PPI	Proton pump inhibitor
PRBC	Packed red blood cells
PRN	As needed, clinical correlation required
PSA	Prostate-specific antigen
PT	Prothrombin time
PTH	Parathyroid hormone
PT/OT	Physical therapy and occupational therapy

(continued)

TABLE GT–1: Abbreviations (Continued)	
PTT	Partial thromboplastin time
PUD	Pelvic ulcer disease
RBC	Red blood cell
r/o	Rule out
RUQ	Right upper quadrant
SBP	Systolic blood pressure
SCD	Sequential compression device
SIMV	Synchronized intermittent mandatory ventilation
SLE	Systemic lupus erythematosus
SOB	Shortness of breath
SPEP	Serum protein electrophoresis
SSRI	Selective serotonin reuptake inhibitor
STD	Sexually transmitted disease
T_3	Thyronine
T_4	Thyroxine
TB	Tuberculosis
TCA	Tricyclic antidepressant
TCP	Transcutaneous pacing
TEE	Transesophageal echocardiogram
TG	Triglyceride
TIA	Transient ischemic attack
TIBC	Total iron binding capacity
TLC	Total lymphocytic count
TMP/SMX	Trimethoprim/sulfamethoxazole
TPN	Total parenteral nutrition
TSH	Thyroid-stimulating hormone
TTE	Transthoracic echocardiogram

(continued)

TABLE GT–1: Abbreviations (Continued)	
TVP	Transvenous pacing
UA	Urine analysis
UC	Ulcerative colitis
Unit	CCU/ICU/SICU/MICU/neuro-ICU
Up ad lib	As tolerated
Urine R&M	Urine random microscopy
URI	Upper respiratory infection
US	Ultrasound
VDRL	Venereal Disease Research Library
VMA	Vanillylmandelic acid
V/Q scan	Ventilation-perfusion scan
WBC	White blood cell
wt	Weight

TABLE GT–2: MIVF	
• First 10 kg of total body wt	• Use 100 mL/kg/day or 4 mL/kg/hr
• Second 10 kg of total body wt	• Use 50 mL/kg/day or 2 mL/kg/hr
• Above 20 kg of total body wt	• Use 20 mL/kg/day or 1 mL/kg/hr

TABLE GT–3: DVT Prophylaxis

Mechanical

- Intermittent pneumatic compression or SCD
- Graduated elastic anti-embolism stockings

Chemical

Medical conditions

- Heparin: 5,000 unit SQ q12h
- Enoxaparin (Lovenox): 40 mg SQ once daily; if CrCl <30 mL/min → 30 mg SQ daily
- Dalteparin (Fragmin): 2,500 units SQ once daily
- Nadroparin:* 2,850 units SQ once daily

General surgery in moderate-risk patient

- Heparin: 5,000 units SQ q12h
- Enoxaparin: 20 mg SQ 1–2 hrs before surgery and daily after surgery
- Dalteparin: 2,500 units SQ 1–2 hrs before surgery and daily after surgery
- Nadroparin:* 2,850 units SQ 2–4 hrs before surgery and daily after surgery
- Tinzaparin (Innohep): 3,500 units SQ 2 hrs before surgery and daily after surgery

General surgery in high-risk patient

- Heparin: 5,000 unit SQ q8h or q12h
- Enoxaparin (Lovenox): 40 mg SQ 1–2 hrs before surgery and daily after surgery or 30 mg SQ q12h starting 8–12 hrs after surgery
- Dalteparin: 5,000 units SQ 8–12 hrs before surgery and daily after surgery

Orthopedic surgery

- Heparin is not recommended

(continued)

TABLE GT–3: DVT Prophylaxis (Continued)
• Enoxaparin: 30 mg SQ q12h starting 12–24 hrs after surgery or 40 mg SQ daily starting 10–12 hrs postsurgery
• Dalteparin: 5,000 units SQ 8–12 hrs before surgery, then daily starting 12–24 hrs after surgery or 2,500 units SQ 6–8 hrs after surgery, then 5,000 units SQ daily
• Nadroparin:* 38 units per kg SQ 12 hrs before surgery; 12 hrs after surgery; and once daily on postoperative days 1, 2, and 3; then ↑ to 57 units per kg SQ daily
• Tinzaparin: 75 units per kg SQ daily starting 12–24 hrs after surgery; or 4,500 units SQ 12 hrs before surgery and daily after surgery
Major trauma
• Heparin: 5,000 unit SQ q8h
• Enoxaparin: 30 mg SQ every 12 hrs (for acute spinal cord injury)
• Enoxaparin: 30 mg SQ every 12 hrs starting 12–36 hrs after injury if the patient is hemodynamically stable
*Not approved.

TABLE GT–4: GI Stress Ulcer Prophylaxis	
H_2 blockers or PPI for following conditions	
• Mechanical ventilation >48 hrs	• >30% burn
• Coagulopathy	• Head trauma
• Shock	• Quadriplegia
• Severe sepsis	• Multiple organ failure
American College of Gastroenterology guidelines for prevention of NSAID–induced ulcer for high-risk conditions	
• Prior GI event	• Age >60 years
• High NSAID dose	• Steroid use
• Anticoagulation	

TABLE GT–5: Bilevel Positive Airway Pressure (BIPAP) Settings*
• **Ventilation**
I (inspiratory positive airway pressure)
Initial: 10–16 cm H_2O
E (expiratory positive airway pressure)
Initial: 3–5 cm H_2O
• **O_2 (oxygenation)**
4–10 L or 50–100%
(Keep <6 L in COPD)
• **RR (respiratory rate)**
Initial: 14–20 breaths per minute
Note
• If CO_2 is high, $\uparrow$ I or $\uparrow$ RR
• If O_2 is low, $\uparrow$ E or $\uparrow$ O_2
*Use requires patient be alert and cooperative.

TABLE GT–6: Initial Ventilator Settings

Settings	Normal	Hypoxic	Obstruction condition	Restrictive lung condition
FiO$_2$	21–100%	100%	40–50%	40–50%
Tidal volume	5–15 L/kg	6 mL/kg	5–7 mL/kg	5–7 mL/kg
RR	12–16 mins	16–24 mins	<24 mins	16–24 mins
Mode	ACV/SIMV	ACV/SIMV	ACV	ACV/SIMV
Positive end-expiratory pressure (PEEP)	Minimal	Variable	PEEP-dependent	FiO$_2$/O$_2$ saturation–dependent
Complications with ventilatory support				
• Barotrauma	• Pneumonia	• DVT		• Neuropathy
• Alveolar overdistention	• Atelectasis	• GI bleed		• Acute sinusitis
• Hypotension				

(continued)

TABLE GT–6: Initial Ventilator Settings (Continued)

Note
• Check CXR after placing patient on ventilator.
• Check ABG in 30 mins to 1 hr after any change in any parameters.
• Hypotension → treat with IVF
• Give DVT and GI prophylaxis to all patients on a ventilator.
• DVT prophylaxis: heparin, 5,000 units SQ bid, or Lovenox, 40 mg SQ daily.
• GI prophylaxis: pantoprazole (Protonix), 40 mg IV daily (bid for GI bleeding)/famotidine (Pepcid), 20 mg IV bid.
• If ABG show high CO_2 → tidal volume can be ↑ to blow off CO_2 *or* ↑ RR.
• PEEP is useful in hypoxic respiratory failure such as acute respiratory distress syndrome or cardiogenic pulmonary edema.
• Low levels of PEEP can be used in chronic obstructive pulmonary disease to keep airways open.
• Increasing PEEP decreases venous return to the heart and might lead to reductions in BP.
• High levels of tidal volume and PEEP might also predispose patients to barotraumas (vent-induced lung injury).

TABLE GT–7: Antibiotic Spectrum

	Gram-positive	Gram-negative	Atypical	Anaerobe	Pseudomonas	Methicillin-resistant *Staphylococcus aureus* (MSSA)	Methicillin-susceptible *S. aureus* (MRSA)
First-generation PCN	+	–	–	–	–	–	–
Second-generation anti-staphylococcus PCN	+	–	–	–	–	–	+
Third-generation amino-PCN	+	±	–	±	–	–	±
Fourth-generation anti-*Pseudomonas* PCN	+	+	–	+	+	–	±
First-generation cephalosporin	+	±	–	–	–	–	+
Second-generation cephalosporin	+	±	–	±	–	–	+

(continued)

TABLE GT–7: Antibiotic Spectrum (Continued)

Third-generation cephalosporin	±	+	−	±	±	−	±
Fourth-generation cephalosporin	+	±	−	±	+	−	±
First-generation quinolones	−	+	−	−	−	−	−
Second-generation quinolones	−	+	±	−	±	−	±
Third-generation quinolones	+	+	+	−	+	−	+
Fourth-generation quinolones	+	+	+	−	±	−	+
Aminoglycoside	−	±	−	−	−	−	+
Macrolide	+	±	+	±	−	−	+
Tetracycline	±	±	+	+	−	±	±
Glycopeptide	+	−	−	±	−	+	+

(continued)

TABLE GT-7: Antibiotic Spectrum (Continued)

Carbapenems	+	+	−	+	±	−	+
Ketolide	+	−	−	±	−	−	+
Miscellaneous							
Aztreonam	−	+	−	−	+	−	−
Daptomycin	+	−	−	−	−	+	+
Linezolid	+	±	±	±	−	+	+
Metronidazole	−	−	−	+	−	−	−

Antibiotic classifications

PCNs

First-generation	Second-generation	Third-generation	Fourth-generation
Benzathine PCN	Dicloxacillin	Amoxicillin	Piperacillin
PCN G benzathine and PCN G procaine (Bicillin C-R)	Nafcillin	Augmentin	Piperacillin/tazobactam (Zosyn)
	Oxacillin	Ampicillin	
PCN G		Unasyn	Timentin

(continued)

TABLE GT–7: Antibiotic Spectrum (Continued)

PCN V				
Procaine PCN			Pivampicillin	
		Cephalosporins		
First-generation	**Second-generation**	**Third-generation**	**Fourth-generation**	
Cefadroxil (Duricef)	Cefaclor (Ceclor)	Cefdinir (Omnicef)	Cefepime (Maxipime)	
Cefazolin (Ancef)	Cefotetan	Cefditoren		
Cephalexin (Keflex)	Cefoxitin	Cefixime (Suprax)		
	Cefprozil	Cefoperazone		
	Cefuroxime	Claforan		
	Loracarbef (Lorabid)	Cefpodoxime		
		Ceftazidime (Fortaz)		
		Ceftizoxime		
		Ceftriaxone (Rocephin)		

(continued)

TABLE GT–7: Antibiotic Spectrum (Continued)

Quinolones

First-generation	Second-generation	Third-generation	Fourth-generation
Nalidixic acid (NegGram)	Ciprofloxacin	Levofloxacin (Levaquin)	Gemifloxacin
	Enoxacin		Moxifloxacin (Avelox)
	Lomefloxacin		
	Norfloxacin		
	Ofloxacin		

Aminoglycosides

Amikacin

Gentamicin

Streptomycin

Tobramycin

Macrolides

Azithromycin (Zithromax)

Clarithromycin (Biaxin)

Dirithromycin (Dynabac)

Erythromycin

Carbapenems

Ertapenem (Invanz)

Imipenem/cilastatin (Primaxin)

Tetracyclines

Doxycycline (Adoxa, Doryx, Monodox)

Minocycline

(continued)

17

TABLE GT-7: Antibiotic Spectrum (Continued)

Meropenem (Merrem)	Tetracycline
Glycopeptide	**Ketolide**
Vancomycin	Telithromycin (Ketek)

Medication peak and trough levels

Medication	Peak	Trough
Amikacin*	20–30 mcg/mL	<10 mcg/mL
Gentamicin (Garamycin)	6–8 mcg/mL	<2 mcg/mL
Streptomycin	15–40 mcg/mL	<5 mcg/mL
Vancomycin (Vancocin)	20–40 mcg/mL (usually not performed)	5–15 mcg/mL (cellulitis)
		10–20 mcg/mL (pneumonia/endocarditis)

Note

- Check vancomycin trough level before third or fourth dose.
- Check gentamicin trough level before fourth dose.

*With amikacin, obtain peak level 30 mins after a 30-min infusion; obtain trough level within 30 mins prior to next dose.

FIGURE GT–1: Dermatomal map.

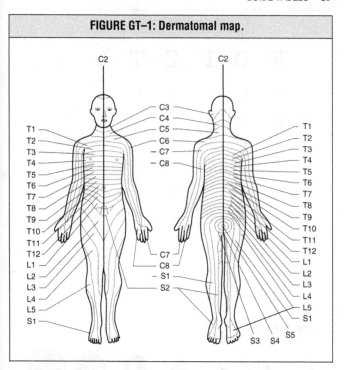

FIGURE GT–2: Near vision testing.

E	O	P	Z	T	L	160 in.
T	D	P	C	F	Z	80 in.
D	Z	E	L	C	F	56 in.
F	E	P	C	T	L	48 in.
P	T	L	F	C	Z	40 in.
E	L	Z	T	C	O	32 in.
D	E	E	L	P	T	24 in.
L	O	P	F	S	E	20 in.
	L	T	C	F	P	16 in.

Hold at 16 in.

Pupil size (mm)

2 3 4 6 8 10 12

1
Cardiology*

---

*See Chapter 5 (Table 5–4) for discussion of endocarditis.

TABLE 1–1: Diagnosis: Chest Pain r/o Acute Coronary Syndrome (ACS)/MI	
Disposition	Unit/cardiac monitored bed
Monitor	Vitals
	Cardiac monitoring
Diet	NPO if procedure planned same day and after midnight if planned next day, ?1- to 2-g sodium diet
Fluid	Heplock (flush every shift)
O$_2$	≥2 L O$_2$ via NC; keep O$_2$ saturation >92%
Activity	Strict bedrest with bedside commode
Dx studies	
Labs	Troponin q8h × 3, CPK-MB q6h × 4, BMP, calcium, Mg, LFT, CBC, PT, PTT, INR, TSH, ?BNP
Radiology and cardiac studies	ECG, CXR (PA and lateral), ?ABG, ?abdominal CT
	If pulmonary embolism (PE) is suspected, spiral CT or V-Q scan, ?venous Doppler of lower extremities
	If aortic dissection suspected, chest CT, cardiac echo [TTE or TEE (preferred)]
Special tests	?Myoglobin stat and q6h (high sensitivity but low specificity), lipid panel, ?toxicology screen
	Exercise stress test (see p. 26), homocysteine level in young patient
Prophylaxis	DVT
Consults	Cardiology

(continued)

TABLE 1–1: Diagnosis: Chest Pain r/o Acute Coronary Syndrome (ACS)/MI (Continued)	
Nursing	Call physician if patient reports of chest pain, stool guaiac
Avoid	Nitroglycerin (NTG) in patient using sildenafil (Viagra)
	Caffeine-containing products
	Pregnancy state: avoid ASA and ACE
	Renal insufficiency or pregnancy: avoid spiral CT
Management	

1. NTG: 0.4 mg SL × 3 q5min [check BP before giving NTG] → if pain not responding to NTG and patient is in severe pain → consider morphine, 2 mg IV q5min.

Note: Hold NTG if SBP <90

2. Nitropaste, 1–1.5 inches, or NTG patch, 0.2 mg/hr q6–8h (off qhs)

3. ASA: 325 mg crushed

4. If chest pain continues despite NTG and morphine → consider NTG drip

NTG drip (mix 100 mg NTG in 500 mL D_5W). **Note:** Hold if SBP <90, heart rate (HR) <60

Give 15-mcg bolus followed by 6 mcg/min (2 mL/hr)

↑ by 6 mcg/min q5min until patient is chest pain–free, SBP <100 (max: 200 mcg/min)

5. Consider enoxaparin (Lovenox): 1 mg/kg bid

6. Metoprolol (Lopressor): 5 mg IV q2–3min × 3 doses, then 25 mg PO q6h; hold if pulse <60 or SBP <90

7. Lorazepam (Ativan): 1–2 mg PO tid–qid PRN for anxiety

8. Consider statin if ↑ lipids: atorvastatin, 10 mg PO qhs, *or* simvastatin, 20 mg PO qhs, *or* pravastatin, 40 mg PO qhs

9. Acetaminophen (Tylenol): 325–650 mg q4–6h PRN for headache

(continued)

TABLE 1–1: Diagnosis: Chest Pain r/o Acute Coronary Syndrome (ACS)/MI (Continued)	
Common etiologies of chest pain	
Emergent	**Nonemergent**
• MI	• GERD
• PE	• Esophageal spasm
• CHF	• Peptic ulcer disease
• Aortic aneurysm	• Hiatal hernia
• Myocarditis/pericarditis	• Herpes zoster
• Tachyarrhythmia	• Mitral valve prolapse
• Pneumonia	• Costochondritis
• Pneumothorax	• Mastitis
• COPD exacerbation	• Thymoma
• Asthma exacerbation	• Lymphoma
• Esophageal rupture	• Anxiety
• Cholecystitis	• Psychoneurosis
• Bowel infarction	• Foreign body
• Pancreatitis	
• Electrolyte abnormalities	
• Diabetic ketoacidosis	

(continued)

TABLE 1–1: Diagnosis: Chest Pain r/o Acute Coronary Syndrome (ACS)/MI (Continued)

Thrombolysis in MI (TIMI) score for UA and non–ST-elevation MI and risk of cardiac events

Criteria	Score	Risk of cardiac events in 14 days (TIMI 11B*)		
		Risk score	Death/MI	Death, MI, or urgent revascularization
Age >65	1			
More than 3 coronary artery disease (CAD) risk factors (HTN, DM, smoker, ↑ cholesterol, FHx of CAD)	1	0/1	3%	5%
Known CAD (stenosis ≥50%)	1	2	3%	8%
ASA use in past 7 days	1	3	5%	13%
Recent severe angina (≤24 hrs)	1	4	7%	20%
↑ Cardiac markers	1	5	12%	26%
ST ↑ ≥0.5 mm	1	6/7	19%	41%

*Entry criteria: UA/non–ST-elevation MI defined as ischemic pain at rest within 24 hrs with evidence of CAD (ST segment deviation or positive marker).

(continued)

TABLE 1–1: Diagnosis: Chest Pain r/o Acute Coronary Syndrome (ACS)/MI (Continued)	
Stress test	
Exercise stress tests	**Imaging study dyes**
1. Treadmill exercise stress test	1. Cardiolite (technetium Tc-99m)
2. Adenosine	Imaging should be performed approximately 1 hr after injecting the dye
Contraindicated in patient with bronchospasm	Long half-life
3. Dobutamine	2. Thallium
Useful in patient with bronchospasm (e.g., COPD, asthma)	Imaging should be performed immediately after injecting the dye
	Short half-life

TABLE 1–2: Diagnosis: Acute Coronary Syndrome (ACS)	
Disposition	Unit
Monitor	Vitals
	Cardiac monitoring
Diet	NPO if procedure planned same day and after midnight if planned next day, ?1- to 2-g sodium diet
Fluid	Heplock (flush every shift)
O_2	≥2 L O_2 via NC; keep O_2 saturation >92%
Activity	Strict bedrest with bedside commode
Dx studies	
Labs	Troponin q8h × 3, CPK-MB q6h × 3, BMP, calcium, Mg, PO_4, LFT, CBC
	UA, PT/PTT/INR, fibrinogen, stool guaiac, fasting lipid panel, TSH
	Urine or serum β-HCG, ?drug toxicology screen (serum/urine)
Radiology and cardiac studies	CXR (PA and lateral), ECG, cardiac echo, exercise stress test
Other tests	?Myoglobin stat and q6h (high sensitivity but low specificity)
	Homocystine level in young patient
Prophylaxis	DVT
Consults	Cardiology
Nursing	Call physician if patient reports of chest pain, stool guaiac
Avoid	Caffeine-containing products
	Patient using Viagra: avoid nitrates
	Pregnancy state: avoid ASA and ACE

(continued)

TABLE 1–2: Diagnosis: Acute Coronary Syndrome (ACS) (Continued)
Management: ACS (non–ST-elevation MI, unstable angina)
1. NTG, 0.4 mg SL × 3 q5min (check BP before giving NTG) → if pain not responding to NTG and patient is in severe pain → consider morphine, 2 mg IV q5min. **Note:** Hold NTG if SBP <90 or pulse <60
2. Nitropaste, 1 inch q8h, or NTG patch, 0.2 mg/hr q12h (off qhs)
3. ASA: 325 mg crushed × 1 PO, then ASA, 162 mg PO daily [if ASA allergy → give clopidogrel (Plavix), 75 mg or 300 mg × 1 dose, then 75 mg PO daily]
4. Consider eptifibatide (Integrilin) IV, bolus of 180 mcg/kg (max: 22.6 mg) over 1–2 mins followed by a continuous infusion of 2 mcg/kg/min (max: 15 mg/hr) up to 72 hrs or up to initiation of coronary artery bypass grafting, or tirofiban (Aggrastat), 0.4 mcg/kg/min × 30 mins, then 0.1 mcg/kg/min × 2–4 days, or abciximab (Reopro), 0.25 mg/kg IV, then 0.125 mcg/kg/min IV infusion × 12 hrs
5. Lopressor: 5 mg IV q2–3min × 3 doses, then 25 mg PO q6h (hold if SBP ≤90 or pulse <60); or atenolol, 5 mg IV, repeated in 5 mins followed by 50–100 mg PO daily; or esmolol, 500 mcg/kg over 1 min, then 50 mcg/kg/min infusion [titrate to pulse >60 bpm (max: 300 mcg/min)]
6. NTG drip (mix 100 mg NTG in 500 mL D_5W). **Note:** Hold if SBP <90, HR <60
Give 15-mcg bolus followed by 6 mcg/min (2 mL/hr)
↑ by 6 mcg/min q5min until patient is chest pain–free, SBP <100 (max: 200 mcg/min)
7. Morphine: 2–4 mg IV push PRN for chest pain not relieved by NTG
8. Lisinopril: 2.5–5 mg PO daily; titrate to 10–20 mg daily
9. Tylenol: 325–650 mg q4–6h PRN for headache
10. Lorazepam (Ativan): 1–2 mg PO tid–qid PRN for anxiety

(continued)

TABLE 1–2: Diagnosis: Acute Coronary Syndrome (ACS) (Continued)
11. Docusate sodium (Colace): 100 mg PO bid for constipation
12. Dimenhydrinate, 25–50 mg IV over 2–5 mins q4–6h or 50 mg PO q4–5h for nausea, *or* ondansetron (Zofran), 2–4 mg IV q4h for N/V
13. Consider statin: atorvastatin, 10 mg PO qhs, *or* simvastatin, 40 mg PO qhs, *or* pravastatin, 40 mg PO qhs
IIb/IIIa dosing for ACS and PCI
• Integrilin: bolus of 180 mcg/kg (max: 22.6 mg) over 1–2 mins, then give 2 mcg/kg/min (max: 15 mg/hr); continue up to 18–24 hrs or until hospital discharge *or*
• Aggrastat: 10 mcg/kg/min, then 0.15 mcg/kg/min × 18–24 hrs *or*
• Abciximab (Reopro): 0.25 mg/kg IV, then 0.125 mcg/kg/min IV infusion × 12–18 hrs

TABLE 1–3: Diagnosis: Acute MI (ST elevation MI)	
Disposition	Unit
Monitor	Vitals
	Cardiac monitoring
Diet	NPO except medication (if possible cardiac catheterization)
	Cardiac diet (low sodium and low fat/low cholesterol)
Fluid	Heplock (flush every shift)
O_2	≥ 2 L O_2 via NC; keep O_2 saturation >92%
Activity	Strict bedrest with bedside commode
Dx studies	
Labs	Troponin q8h × 3, CPK-MB q6h × 3, CBC, BMP, calcium, Mg, PO_4, LFT
	PT/INR/PTT, TSH, fasting lipid panel, UA, fibrinogen
Radiology and cardiac studies	CXR (PA and lateral), ECG in 12 hrs × 2, cardiac echo, ?cardiac catheterization
Special tests	?Myoglobin stat and then q6h (high sensitivity but low specificity)
	Urine or serum β-HCG, homocysteine level in young patient
	?Drug toxicology screen (serum/urine)
Prophylaxis	?
Consults	Cardiology
Nursing	Call physician if patient reports of chest pain, stool guaiac
Avoid	Patient using Viagra: avoid using NTG
	Pregnancy state: avoid ACE and ASA
Management	See Management: Acute MI; also see thrombolytic therapy criteria

(continued)

FIGURE 1–1: ST elevation MI.

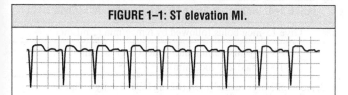

TABLE 1–3: Diagnosis: Acute MI (ST elevation MI) (Continued)		
ECG Leads and Arterial Supply Associations		
ECG leads	**Blood vessel**	**Area supplied**
V1–V4	LAD coronary artery	Anterior
V5–V6	Left circumflex	Lateral
I, aVL, V4–V6	Left circumflex	Lateral
II, III, and aVF	RCA	Inferior
R/S ratio >1 in V1–V2 and reciprocal T inversion in V1	Distal circumflex, posterior descending, or distal RCA	Posterior
I, aVL, V5, and V6	Diagonal branch of LAD coronary artery, marginal branch of left circumflex, left circumflex	Anterolateral
V1–V3	LAD coronary artery	Anteroseptal
Management: Acute MI		
1. NTG: 0.4 mg SL × 3 q5min (check BP before giving NTG) → if pain not responding to NTG and patient is in severe pain → consider morphine, 2 mg IV q5min (hold NTG if SBP <90) *or*		
2. NTG ointment: 1–1.5 inches, or NTG patch, 0.2–0.6 mg/hr q6–8h off qhs (hold NTG if SBP <90) *or*		
NTG drip (mix 100 mg NTG in 500 mL D_5W). **Note:** Hold if SBP <90, HR <60		

(continued)

TABLE 1–3: Diagnosis: Acute MI (ST elevation MI) (Continued)
Give 15-mcg bolus followed by 6 mcg/min (2 mL/hr)
↑ by 6 mcg/min q5min until patient is chest pain–free, SBP <100 (max: 200 mcg/min)
3. ASA, 325 mg crushed, then 162 mg EC PO daily ± Plavix, 75 mg or 300 mg × 1 dose, then 75 mg PO daily
4. Consider thrombolytic (alteplase or reteplase) if patient presents within 12 hrs (check stool guaiac)
5. Consider integrelin with ACS (non–Q-wave MI and unstable angina) or with planned PCI
6. Lopressor: 5 mg IV q2–3min × 3 doses, then 25 mg PO q6h (hold if SBP ≤90 or HR <60) *or*
Atenolol: 5 mg IV, repeated in 5 mins followed by 50–100 mg PO daily (hold if SBP ≤90 or HR <60) *or*
Esmolol: 500 mcg/kg over 1 min, then 50 mcg/kg/min infusion (hold if SBP ≤90 or HR <60)
7. Heparin drip: 80–100 unit/kg bolus, then 18–20 unit/kg or 1,000 unit/hr (check stool guaiac before r/o bleeding)
Check PT/PTT, which should be 1.5–2 times the control, and check 6 hrs after
Patient can be started on Lovenox, mainly for unstable angina or non–Q-wave MI at 1 mg/kg SQ bid instead of heparin (adjust dose in renal failure: if CrCl <30 mL/min, use 1 mg/kg q24h)
8. Morphine: 2–4 mg IV push PRN for chest pain not relieved by NTG × 3
9. Consider ACE (lisinopril, 2.5–5 mg PO daily; titrate to 10–20 mg daily)
10. Lorazepam (Ativan): 1–2 mg PO tid–qid PRN for anxiety
11. Tylenol: 325–650 mg q4–6h PRN for headache
12. Consider atorvastatin, 10 mg PO qhs, *or* simvastatin, 40 mg PO qhs, *or* pravastatin, 40 mg PO qhs (consider high-dose statin)

(continued)

TABLE 1–3: Diagnosis: Acute MI (ST elevation MI) (Continued)
13. Colace, 100 mg PO bid for constipation
14. Dimenhydrinate, 25–50 mg IV over 2–5 mins q4–6h or 50 mg PO q4–5h for N/V, *or* Zofran, 2–4 mg IV q4h for N/V
Note
• If heparin-induced thrombocytopenia present, consider argatroban, 2 mcg/kg/min IV continuous infusion
Max 10 mcg/kg/min, adjust until steady-state aPTT is 1.5–3 times baseline value
• Avoid using NTG in patients using Viagra and ACE and ASA in pregnant patients
• Patients with unstable angina should be started on Lovenox, 1 mg/kg bid
• EF <40%, patient should be on ACE/ARB/hydralazine and nitrate
• Be cautious of starting heparin in patient with history of cancer due to risk of bleeding
Criteria for fibrinolytic therapy
• Onset of symptoms ≤3 hrs can be given up to 12 hrs (most beneficial if given within 30 mins)
• ST segment ↑ of >1 mm in two or more contiguous ECG limb leads *or*
• A new left bundle branch block
Absolute contraindications to fibrinolytic therapy
• Prior intracranial hemorrhage
• Documented structural cerebral vascular lesion (e.g., AVM)
• Documented intracranial malignant tumor (primary or metastatic)
• Ischemic stroke within 3 mos with exception of acute ischemic stroke within 3 hrs

(continued)

TABLE 1-3: Diagnosis: Acute MI (ST elevation MI) (Continued)
• Active bleeding or bleeding diathesis (does not include menses)
• Suspected aortic dissection
• Significant closed-head or facial trauma within 3 mos
Relative contraindications to fibrinolytic therapy
• History of chronic, severe, poorly controlled HTN
• Severe uncontrolled HTN (SBP >180 or DBP >110)
• History of prior ischemic stroke >3 mos, dementia, or documented intracranial pathology
• Active peptic ulcer
• Pregnancy
• Traumatic or prolonged CPR (>10 mins) or major surgery within <3 weeks
• Recent internal bleeding (2–4 weeks)
• Noncompressible vascular punctures

TABLE 1–4: Diagnosis: CHF	
Disposition	Unit
Monitor	Vitals
	Cardiac monitoring
	Electrolyte monitoring (mainly K^+)
Diet	Low salt (1- to 2-g) diet, cardiac diet, and fluid restriction 1,200–1,600 mL
	?NPO
Fluid	Heplock (flush every shift)
O_2	$\geq$2 L O_2 via NC; keep O_2 saturation >92%
Activity	Strict bedrest with bedside commode
Dx studies	
Labs	Troponin q8h $\times$ 3, CPK-MB q6h $\times$ 4, BNP, BMP
	Calcium, Mg, PO_4, LFT, CBC, PT/PTT/INR, fasting lipid panel, TSH level, UA
Radiology and cardiac studies	CXR (PA and lateral), ECG, cardiac echo, ?impedance cardiography
Special tests	?Myoglobin stat and then q6h (high sensitivity but low specificity)
	?Serial BNP, iron studies
Prophylaxis	DVT
	Antiembolism stocking to control lower extremity edema
	Influenza (flu) and pneumococcal vaccine
Consults	Cardiology
Nursing	I/O, daily weight, head of bed and legs elevated, Foley catheter
	Stool guaiac

(continued)

TABLE 1–4: Diagnosis: CHF (Continued)	
Avoid	• NSAIDs, pseudoephedrine-containing products (i.e., nasal decongestants)
	• Diastolic dysfunction: avoid vigorous diuresis to maintain CO
	• Aortic stenosis: avoid ACE in severe aortic stenosis; use nitrates with precautions
	• IHSS: avoid vigorous diuresis, digitalis, ACE, and hydralazine
	• Avoid using ACE and ASA in pregnancy; consider avoiding NSAIDs, nasal decongestants
Management	
1. Loop diuretics	
If loop diuretics ineffective → add metolazone (Zaroxolyn), 5–10 mg PO daily	
Spironolactone: add to poorly compensated cases [useful in New York class III–IV heart failure (*N Engl J Med* 341, 10:709–717)]	
2. KCl: 20–60 mEq PO daily if patient on loop diuretic	
3. Nesiritide (Natrecor): useful in decompensated CHF and low EF	
Natrecor preparation: add 1.5 mg in 250 mL D_5W → dilution concentration: 6 mcg/mL	
Bolus: 2 mcg/kg; infusion rate: 0.01 mcg/kg/min (contraindicated if SBP <100) *or*	
NTG: 5 mcg/min IV infusion, ↑ at rate of 5 mcg/min (hold if SBP <90) (50 mg in 250 mL D_5W)	
4. Morphine: 2–4 mg IV push PRN for anxiety	
5. ACE: check CrCl (see below)	
If ACE contraindicated → consider ARB or hydralazine + isosorbide	

(continued)

TABLE 1–4: Diagnosis: CHF (Continued)

6. Digoxin: if patient has atrial fibrillation or severe CHF, or EF <30% → start at 0.5–1 mg IV/PO × 1 dose followed by 0.25 mg IV × 2 doses, then 0.125–0.25 mg daily

7. β-Blocker: Hold if ↓ BP or ↓ pulse

Most proven is carvedilol, 3.125 mg PO bid × 2 weeks, then 6.25 mg PO bid × 2 weeks *or*

Bisoprolol (Zebeta): 5–20 mg/day [decreases all-cause mortality and morbidity in CIBIS-II study (*Lancet* 1999, 352, 9–13)]

Note: Be cautious of using β-blockers in patient with COPD.

8. Dopamine: 3–15 mcg/kg/min IV; titrate to CO >4, CI >2, SBP >90

(400 mg in 250 mL D_5W → 1,600 mcg/mL) *or*

Dobutamine: 2.5–10 mcg/kg/min IV; max: 14 mcg/kg/min (500 mg in 250 mL D_5W → 2 mcg/mL) *or*

Milrinone: 0.375 mcg/kg/min IV infusion; titrate to 0.75 mcg/kg/min (side effects: arrhythmia and hypotension)

9. ASA: 81 mg PO daily, *or* Plavix, 75 mg PO daily, if associated CAD

10. Warfarin (Coumadin): (5–10 mg to keep INR 2–3) if EF <30%

11. Colace: 100 mg PO bid for constipation

12. Dimenhydrinate: 25–50 mg IV over 2–5 mins q4–6h or 50 mg PO q4–5h for nausea, *or* Zofran, 2–4 mg IV q4h for N/V

Commonly Used Medications in CHF		
	Initial dose	**Max dose**
Loop diuretics		
Bumetanide	0.5–1 mg daily–bid	Titrate to achieve dry weight (up to 10 mg daily)
Furosemide	20–60 mg daily–bid	Titrate to achieve dry weight (up to 400 mg daily)

(continued)

TABLE 1–4: Diagnosis: CHF (Continued)		
	Initial dose	**Max dose**
Torsemide	10–20 mg daily–bid	Titrate to achieve dry weight (up to 200 mg daily)
ACE inhibitors		
Captopril	6.25 mg tid	50 mg tid
Enalapril	2.5 mg bid	10–20 mg bid
Fosinopril	5–10 mg daily	40 mg daily
Lisinopril	2.5–5 mg daily	20–40 mg daily
Quinapril	10 mg daily	40 mg bid
Ramipril	1.25–2.5 mg daily	10 mg daily
β-Blockers		
Bisoprolol	1.25 mg daily	10 mg daily
Carvedilol	3.125 mg bid	25 mg bid; if weight >85 kg → 50 mg bid
Metoprolol tartrate	6.25 mg bid	75 mg bid
Metoprolol succinate	12.5–25 mg daily	200 mg daily
Digitalis glycosides		
Digoxin	0.125–0.25 mg daily	0.125–0.25 mg daily
Note: Monitor potassium when using loop diuretic and keep potassium >4.		
Source: From American Heart Association.		

TABLE 1–5: Diagnosis: Hypertensive Emergency (See BP Classification)	
Disposition	Cardiac-monitored bed/unit
Monitor	Vitals, BP check q30min, then q2–4h once BP is stable
	Cardiac monitoring
	Neuromonitoring
Diet	?Clear liquids, ?heart healthy, ?low sodium
Fluid	Heplock (flush every shift)
O_2	≥2 L O_2 via NC; keep O_2 saturation >92%
Activity	Strict bedrest with bedside commode
Dx studies	
Labs	CBC, BMP, calcium, LFT, UA, urine R&M, TSH, troponin q8h × 3
	CPK-MB q6h × 4, fasting lipid profile, drug toxicology screen (serum/urine), uric acid
Radiology and cardiac studies	?Myoglobin stat and then q6h (high sensitivity but low specificity)
	CXR (PA and lateral), ?cardiac echo (aortic aneurysm), ?head CT, ECG
	If intracranial hemorrhage is suspected → head CT or LP
	If renal artery stenosis is suspected → renal ultrasound, intraarterial angiography
	?Impedance cardiography
Special tests	?Catecholamine, ?24-hr catecholamine, ?24-hr urine metanephrine and VMA
	?Renin level, ?aldosterone level, funduscopy
Prophylaxis	DVT

(continued)

TABLE 1–5: Diagnosis: Hypertensive Emergency (See BP Classification) (Continued)	
	Constipation and coughing prophylaxis to prevent intracranial bleeding
Consults	Cardiology, nephrology
Nursing	I/O, urine output, daily weights, stool guaiac
Avoid	ASA, Plavix, caffeine-containing products
Management	See Management: BP

High BP Signs and Symptoms

Life-threatening conditions	Signs and symptoms
• Hypertensive encephalopathy	• Headache, blurry vision
• MI	• Chest pain (may not have chest pain in elderly/diabetes mellitus)
• Aortic dissection	• Back pain, chest pain
• Neurologic	• Sensory or motor loss, altered mental status
• Arterial thrombus	• Peripheral pulses
• Renal	• ↓ urine output
• Eclampsia in pregnancy	• Seizure, convulsions

BP Classification

	Uncontrolled HTN	Urgency	Emergency
BP	>180/110	>180/110	>220/140
Signs and symptoms	Headache	Severe headache	Chest pain, SOB
	Anxiety	SOB	Dysarthria
	Asymptomatic	Edema	Altered consciousness

(continued)

TABLE 1–5: Diagnosis: Hypertensive Emergency (See BP Classification) (Continued)			
	Uncontrolled HTN	**Urgency**	**Emergency**
			Encephalopathy
			Pulmonary edema
			CVA
			Cardiac ischemia

Management: BP			
	Dosage	**Onset**	**Duration**
PO agents			
Clonidine	0.1–0.2 mg initially, then 0.1 mg q1h up to 0.8	30–60 mins	6–8 hrs
Captopril	12.5–25 mg PO tid (may cause hypotension)	15–30 mins	4–6 hrs
Labetalol	200–400 mg PO daily q2–3h	30 mins–2 hrs	2–12 hrs
Prazosin	1–2 mg PO q1h	1–2h	8–12 hrs
IV agents			
Nitroprusside	Drip 50 mg in 250 mL D_5W; start at 3 mcg/kg/min; max: 10 mcg/kg/min (check thiocyanate level)	Seconds	3–5 mins
	Use **caution** when nitroprusside used >24 hrs, especially in renal failure		

(continued)

TABLE 1–5: Diagnosis: Hypertensive Emergency (See BP Classification) (Continued)			
	Dosage	**Onset**	**Duration**
Esmolol	5 g in 500 mL D$_5$W, loading dose of 500 mcg/kg over 1 min, then 50–200 mcg/kg/min	1–2 mins	10–30 mins
Trimethaphan	0.5–5 mg/min (useful in aortic dissection)	1–3 mins	10 mins
Nicardipine	5 mg/hr; ↑ by 1–2.5 mg/hr q15min, max: 15 mg/hr	1–5 mins	3–6 hrs
NTG	0.25–5 mcg/kg/min; patient may develop tolerance	2–5 mins	3–5 mins
Fenoldopam	0.1–1.6 mcg/mg/min; may protect renal function	4–5 mins	<10 mins
Hydralazine	5–20 mg q20min IV (side effect: headache)	10–30 mins	2–6 hrs
Labetalol	Start at 20 mg → 40 mg → 60 mg → 80 mg; repeat every 10–15 mins, max: up to 300 mg	5–10 mins	3–6 hrs
Furosemide	10–80 mg (use in conjunction with vasodilator)	15 mins	4 hrs
Enalapril (Vasotec)	1.25–2.5 mg q6h (max: 5 mg/24 hrs); may continue as PO	15 mins	>6 hrs

(continued)

	Dosage	Onset	Duration
	Caution: ↓ dose if CrCl <30, Cr >3, or renal stenosis		

TABLE 1–5: Diagnosis: Hypertensive Emergency (See BP Classification) (Continued)

Maintenance BP management

- Labetalol, 200–600 mg PO bid (max: 2,400 mg/day)

- Lopressor, 50–100 mg PO daily

- Hydralazine, 25–50 mg PO bid–qid

- Nicardipine, 30–60 mg PO bid (max: 120 mg/day)

Note

- Labetalol not recommended for patients with asthma, COPD, CHF, heart block, bradycardia, cardiogenic shock

- Nitroprusside not recommended in pregnancy

- Hydralazine recommended in pregnancy

- CNS symptoms: avoid centrally acting medications, use β-blockers

TABLE 1–6: Diagnosis: Hypotension	
Disposition	Unit
Monitor	Vitals
	Cardiac monitoring
	Electrolyte monitoring
	Neuromonitoring
Diet	PRN
Fluid	Wide open initially (caution in patient with CHF)
O_2	≥2 L O_2 via NC; keep O_2 saturation >92%
Activity	Bedrest
Dx studies	
Labs	CBC with differential, BMP, calcium, Mg, PO_4, LFT, amylase, lipase, TSH
	Troponin q8h × 3, CPK-MB q6h × 4, ABG
	Fibrin split product, fibrinogen, lactic acid
Radiology and cardiac studies	ECG, CXR (PA and lateral), abdominal x-ray (r/o obstruction), ?abdominal CT
	?Pulmonary artery catheterization to determine etiology
Special tests	?Myoglobin stat and then q6h
	?Blood C&S, ?type and cross PRBC, serum/urine toxicology screen
	Serum/urine toxicology screen, ?cortisol level
Prophylaxis	DVT
Consults	Cardiology
Nursing	Trendelenburg position, stool guaiac, I/O, Foley catheter, low bed

(continued)

TABLE 1–6: Diagnosis: Hypotension (Continued)	
Avoid	Antihypertensive medications

Management
• Epinephrine (Levophed): ACLS dosing range of 0.5–30 mcg/min *or* mix 4 mg in 500 mL D_5W
• Initially: 4 mcg/min = 30 mL/hr; usual range: 8–12 mcg/min
• Microgram to mL comparison according to mixture of 4 mg in 500 mL
4 mcg/min = 30 mL/hr
6 mcg/min = 45 mL/hr
8 mcg/min = 60 mL/hr
10 mcg/min = 75 mL/hr
• Dopamine dosing: max: 50 mcg/kg/min; nonrenal property starts at >15 mcg/kg/min
• Premixed in D_5W
0.8 mg/mL in 250 mL or 500 mL
1.6 mg/mL in 250 mL or 500 mL
3.2 mg/mL in 250 mL

TABLE 1–7: Diagnosis: Asystole	
Disposition	?
Monitor	Vitals
	Cardiac monitoring
	Electrolyte monitoring
	Neuromonitoring
Diet	NPO
Fluid	Heplock
O$_2$	PRN
Activity	Bedrest
Dx studies	
Labs	CBC, BMP, Mg, PO$_4$, PT/PTT/INR, LFT, ABG, serum toxicology screen, troponin q8h
Radiology and cardiac studies	CXR (PA and lateral), ECG
Prophylaxis	?
Consults	Check code status
Nursing	Pulse oximetry
Avoid	?
Management	See Management: Asystole

(continued)

FIGURE 1–2: Asystole.

TABLE 1–7: Diagnosis: Asystole (Continued)

Management: Asystole

- Check for code status before starting CPR
- Check ABCs
- Check pulse
- If no pulse, start CPR
- Check vitals
- Consider transcutaneous pacing
- Epinephrine, 1 mg IV q3–5min
- Atropine, 1 mg IV q3–5min (max: 0.04 mg/kg)
- If asystole persists, consider withholding resuscitation

Note: Always confirm asystole in two perpendicular leads. Also need to consider isoelectric V-fib.

Source: From American Heart Association.

TABLE 1–8: Diagnosis: Bradycardia	
Disposition	Unit
Monitor	Vitals
	Cardiac monitoring
Diet	?NPO
Fluid	IVF (?wide open–?MIVF)
O₂	≥ 2 L O_2 via NC; keep O_2 saturation >92%
Activity	Bedrest
Dx studies	
Labs	CBC, BMP, calcium, Mg, PO₄, LFT, TSH, troponin q8h × 3, CPM-MB q6h × 4
Radiology and cardiac studies	CXR (PA and lateral), ECG, ?cardiac echo, event monitor, ?Holter monitor
	?Electrophysiological study, ?exercise stress test
Special tests	?Myoglobin stat and then q6h (high sensitivity but low specificity)
	?Troponin q8h, ?serum/urine toxicology screen, digoxin levels if patient already on digoxin
Prophylaxis	DVT
Consults	Cardiology
Nursing	Atropine at bedside
Avoid	β-Blockers, digoxin, amiodarone, clonidine, diltiazem, verapamil
	Note: Do not use lidocaine to treat escape slow wide complex rhythm
Management	See Management: Bradycardia

(continued)

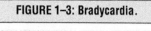

FIGURE 1–3: Bradycardia.

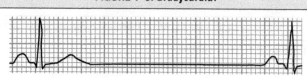

TABLE 1–8: Diagnosis: Bradycardia (Continued)
Management: Bradycardia
Symptomatic
• Place patient in Trendelenburg position
• Atropine: 0.5–1 mg IV push q3–5min (max: 0.04 mg/kg)
• Then consider TCP
• If NR, dopamine, 5–20 mcg/kg/min
• If NR, epinephrine, 2–10 mcg/min
• If NR, isoproterenol, 2–10 mcg/min
Asymptomatic
• If second-degree type II or third-degree heart block → consider TCP or TVP
• For all other AV blocks or sinus node dysfunction → have atropine at bedside
• When patient becomes symptomatic, follow above symptomatic protocol
Source: From American Heart Association.

TACHYARRHYTHMIA

TABLE 1–9A: Diagnosis: Atrial Fibrillation/Atrial Flutter
Treatment for rate control
• Diltiazem (Cardizem): 20 mg IV over 2 mins, re-bolus in 15 mins, *or*
• Esmolol: 500 mcg/kg IV over 1 min, *or*
• Verapamil, 2.5–5 mg IV initially then 5–10 mg IV, *or*
• Lopressor, 50 mg PO
• If low EF/low BP → digoxin, 0.5 mg IV bolus, then 0.25 mg IV q2h until rate is controlled (max:1.5 mg)
Treatment for maintenance of sinus rhythm
• Procainamide, 2–6 mg/kg IV over 5 mins followed by 20–80 mcg/kg/min infusion (max: 2 g/day), *or*
• Amiodarone (for impaired ventricular function) *or*
• Ibutilide *or*
• Flecainide *or*
• Propafenone *or*
• **Direct current** cardioversion if medical therapy fails or patient is symptomatic
• **Anticoagulation is recommended** unless there is a contraindication
Note
• Consider placing patient on Cardizem drip; start at 5 mg/hr titrate for rate control
• Consider anticoagulant with heparin and then Coumadin
• Urgent cardioversion: start heparin IV stat, then check TEE, then cardiovert within 24 hrs, then anticoagulate for 4 more weeks
• Delayed cardioversion: anticoagulate for at least 3 weeks (keep INR 2–3), then cardiovert, then anticoagulate for 4 more weeks

FIGURE 1–4: Atrial fibrillation.

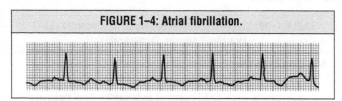

FIGURE 1–5: Atrial flutter.

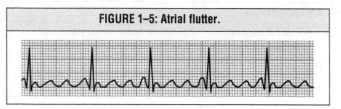

TABLE 1–9B: Diagnosis: Supraventricular Tachycardia (SVT) (Narrow-Complex Tachycardia)	
Atrial tachycardia	
Atrial fibrillation/atrial flutter, MAT, sinus/inappropriate tachycardia, sinus nodal reentrant tachycardia, atrial tachycardia	
AV tachycardia	
AV nodal reentrant or AV reentrant tachycardia, junctional ectopic tachycardia, paroxysmal junctional tachycardia	
Disposition	Unit
Monitor	Vitals
	Cardiac monitoring
Diet	?NPO, cardiac diet, low fat, low cholesterol, no caffeine
Fluid	Heplock (flush every shift)
O_2	≥2 L O_2 via NC; keep O_2 saturation >92%
Activity	Bedrest
Dx studies	
Labs	CBC, BMP, calcium, Mg, PO_4, LFT, PT/INR/PTT, TSH, UA, troponin q8h × 3
	CPK-MB q6h × 3
Radiology and cardiac studies	CXR (PA and lateral), ECG, cardiac echo (TEE)
Special tests	?Myoglobin stat and then q6h (high sensitivity but low specificity)
	?Serum/urine toxicology screen, digoxin levels if patient already on digoxin
Prophylaxis	DVT
Consults	Cardiology
Nursing	Stool guaiac

(continued)

TABLE 1–9B: Diagnosis: Supraventricular Tachycardia (SVT) (Narrow-Complex Tachycardia) (Continued)	
Avoid	Caffeine-containing products
Management	See Management: SVT (Narrow-Complex Tachycardia)

FIGURE 1–6: SVT.

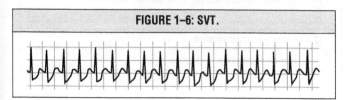

Management: SVT (Narrow-Complex Tachycardia)

- If patient is unstable → cardiovert

- Vagal maneuver/carotid massage → NR → adenosine, 6 mg → NR → 12 mg → NR→ 12 mg → Cardizem, 15–20 mg (0.25 mg/kg) IV over 2 mins → NR after 15 mins → 20–25 mg over 2 mins

- Check the rhythm

- If junctional tachycardia (can be caused by digoxin or theophylline overdose)

  If normal EF → β-blocker, calcium channel blocker, amiodarone

  If EF <40%, CHF → amiodarone

- If multifocal atrial tachycardia (commonly seen in COPD patients)

  Correct hypoxemia first

  If normal EF → β-blocker, calcium channel blocker, amiodarone

  If EF <40%, CHF → amiodarone

(continued)

TABLE 1–9B: Diagnosis: Supraventricular Tachycardia (SVT) (Narrow-Complex Tachycardia) (Continued)
• If PSVT
If normal EF → β-blocker, calcium channel blocker, digoxin → **direct current** cardioversion
Also consider procainamide, amiodarone, or sotalol
If EF <40% → digoxin → NR → amiodarone → NR → diltiazem
If unstable → cardioversion
Source: From American Heart Association.

TABLE 1–9C: Diagnosis: Ventricular Tachycardia (VT) (Wide-Complex Tachycardia)	
Disposition	Unit
Monitor	Vitals
	Cardiac monitoring
Diet	?NPO, cardiac diet, low fat, low cholesterol, no caffeine
Fluid	Heplock (flush every shift)
O$_2$	≥2 L O$_2$ via NC; keep O$_2$ saturation >92%
Activity	Bedrest
Dx studies	
Labs	CBC, BMP, calcium, Mg, PO$_4$, LFT, PT/INR/PTT, TSH, UA
	Troponin q8h × 3, CPK-MB q6h × 3
Radiology and cardiac studies	CXR (PA and lateral), ECG, ?cardiac echo
Special tests	?Myoglobin stat and then q6h (high sensitivity but low specificity)
	?Serum/urine toxicology screen, signal-averaged ECG
Prophylaxis	DVT
Consults	Cardiology
Nursing	None
Avoid	β-Blocker, calcium channel blocker, digoxin, caffeine-containing products
Management	See Management: VT (Wide-Complex Tachycardia), Stable

(continued)

FIGURE 1–7: Ventricular tachycardia.

TABLE 1–9C: Diagnosis: Ventricular Tachycardia (VT) (Wide-Complex Tachycardia) (Continued)

Management: VT (Wide-Complex Tachycardia), Stable

Monomorphic → may consider synchronized cardioversion

- If EF <55% → amiodarone, 150 mg IV/10 mins, or lidocaine, 0.5–0.75 mg/kg, then cardioversion

- If EF >55% → procainamide load, 20 mg/min up to 17 mg/kg (1,000 mg), then infuse 1–4 mg/min (max: 17 mg/kg)

or

Procainamide, 100 mg IV over 5 mins q10min when effective; maintain IV rate at 2 mg/min

Also consider sotalol, amiodarone, lidocaine

Polymorphic → search for electrolyte abnormality (K, Mg), drug toxicity, ischemia

- Normal QT:

If EF <55% → amiodarone, 150 mg IV/10 mins, *or* lidocaine, 0.5–0.75 mg/kg

If EF >55% → β-blocker, lidocaine, amiodarone, sotalol

If NR → synchronized cardioversion

- Prolonged QT (suggestive of torsades) → Mg, overdrive pacing, isoproterenol, phenytoin, lidocaine

Source: From American Heart Association.

TABLE 1–9D: Diagnosis: Ventricular Fibrillation (V-Fib)/Unstable VT	
Disposition	Unit
Monitor	Vitals
	Cardiac monitoring
Diet	?NPO, cardiac diet, low fat, low cholesterol, no caffeine
Fluid	Heplock (flush every shift)
O$_2$	≥2 L O$_2$ via NC; keep O$_2$ saturation >92%
Activity	Bedrest
Dx studies	
Labs	CBC, BMP, calcium, Mg, PO$_4$, LFT, PT/INR/PTT, TSH, UA
	Troponin q8h × 3, CPK-MB q6h × 8
Radiology and cardiac studies	CXR (PA and lateral), ECG, ?cardiac echo
Special tests	?Myoglobin stat and then q6h (high sensitivity but low specificity)
	?Serum/urine toxicology screen, signal-averaged ECG
Prophylaxis	DVT
Consults	Cardiology
Nursing	?
Avoid	Caffeine-containing products
Management	See Management: V-Fib/Unstable VT

(continued)

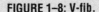

FIGURE 1–8: V-fib.
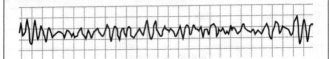

TABLE 1–9D: Diagnosis: Ventricular Fibrillation (V-Fib)/Unstable VT (Continued)
Management: V-Fib/Unstable VT
• Start CPR (consider placing patient on ventilator)
• Precordial thump if no defibrillator immediately available
• Shock 200 J → NR → shock 200–300 J → and then 360 J
• If NR → epinephrine, 1 mg IV q3–5min, *or* vasopressin, 40U IV × 1 dose
• If NR → shock 360 J → NR → amiodarone, 300 mg IV, then give 150 mg in 3–5 mins (max: 2.2 g IV/24 hrs)
• If NR → shock 360 J → lidocaine, 1–1.5 mg/kg IV [may repeat in 3–5 mins (max: 3 mg/kg)]
• If NR → shock 360 J → magnesium sulfate, 1–2 g IV **push** over 2 mins (for hypomagnesemia/torsades de pointes)
• If NR → shock 360 J → procainamide, 30 mg/min or 100 mg IV q5min up to 17 mg/kg
• If NR → shock 360 J → HCO_3, 1 mEq/kg IV
• If NR → shock 360 J
Note: If patient has pacemaker, start shock at >200 J
Source: From American Heart Association.

TABLE 1–9E: Diagnosis: WPW Syndrome (Short P-R, Narrow-Complex Tachycardia, Delta Wave)	
Disposition	Cardiac-monitored bed/unit
Monitor	Vitals
	Cardiac monitoring
Diet	?NPO, cardiac diet, low fat, low cholesterol, no caffeine
Fluid	Heplock (flush every shift)
O_2	≥ 2 L O_2 via NC; keep O_2 saturation >92%
Activity	Bedrest
Dx studies	
Labs	CBC, BMP, calcium, Mg, PO_4, LFT, PT/INR/PTT, TSH, UA
	Troponin q8h × 3, CPK-MB q6h × 4
Radiology and cardiac studies	CXR (PA and lateral), ECG, ?cardiac echo
Special tests	?Myoglobin stat and then q6h (high sensitivity but low specificity)
	?Serum/urine toxicology screen, signal-averaged ECG
Prophylaxis	DVT
Consults	Cardiology
Nursing	?
Avoid	Digoxin, β-blocker, calcium channel blocker, and adenosine; caffeine-containing products

(continued)

FIGURE 1–9: WPW syndrome.

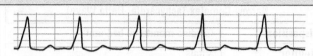

TABLE 1–9E: Diagnosis: WPW Syndrome (Short P-R, Narrow-Complex Tachycardia, Delta Wave) (Continued)
Management
Delta wave is −VE in V1, V2, and aVR; +VE in I, II, aVL, and aVF; and isoelectric in III
Treatment if EF normal
• Direct current cardioversion *or*
Amiodarone: 150 mg IV over 10 mins and repeat q10min, *or*
Procainamide: load 20 mg/min up to 17 mg/kg (1,000 mg), then infuse 1–4 mg/min (max: 17 mg/kg) *or*
Procainamide: 100 mg IV over 5 mins q10min; when WPW resolves, maintain IV rate at 2 mg/min
• Flecainide *or*
Propafenone *or*
Sotalol
Treatment if EF <40% or CHF
• Direct current cardioversion *or*
Amiodarone: 150 mg IV over 10 mins and repeat q10min
Note
• If duration of WPW >48 hrs → consider anticoagulation
• Urgent cardioversion: start heparin IV stat, then check TEE, then cardiovert within 24 hrs, then anticoagulate for 4 more weeks
• Delayed cardioversion: anticoagulate for at least 3 weeks (keep INR 2–3), then cardiovert, then anticoagulate for 4 more weeks

Source: From American Heart Association.

TABLE 1–9F: Diagnosis: Torsades de Pointes		
Disposition	Cardiac-monitored bed/unit	
Monitor	Vitals	
	Cardiac monitoring	
Diet	?NPO, cardiac diet, low fat, low cholesterol, no caffeine	
Fluid	Heplock (flush every shift)	
O_2	≥2 L O_2 via NC; keep O_2 saturation >92%	
Activity	Bedrest	
Dx studies		
Labs	CBC, BMP, calcium, Mg, PO_4, LFT, PT/INR/PTT, TSH, UA	
	Troponin q8h × 3, CPK-MB q6h × 4	
Radiology and cardiac studies	?Myoglobin stat and then q6h (high sensitivity but low specificity)	
	CXR (PA and lateral), ECG, ?cardiac echo	
Special tests	?Serum/urine toxicology screen	
Prophylaxis	DVT	
Consults	Cardiology	
Nursing	?	
Avoid	Amiodarone	Ketoconazole
	Bepridil	Moricizine
	Disopyramide	Phenothiazine
	Haloperidol	Procainamide
	Hypokalemia	Procainamide
	Hypokalemia	Sotalol
	Hypomagnesemia	Tetracycline
	Ibutilide	TCAs

(continued)

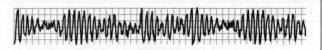

FIGURE 1–10: Torsades de pointes.

TABLE 1–9F: Diagnosis: Torsades de Pointes (Continued)

Management

- Polymorphic VT plus QT prolongation

- Magnesium sulfate: 1–4 g IV bolus over 5–15 mins, *or*

  Magnesium sulfate: 2–20 mg/min IV infusion; max: up to 48 hrs
  until QTc interval <440 msecs

- Isoproterenol: 12–20 mcg/min (2 mg in 500 mL $D_5W \rightarrow$ 4 mcg/mL)

- If medical treatment fails → consider overdrive ventricular
  pacing or cardioversion

TABLE 1–9G: Diagnosis: Pulseless Electric Activity	
Disposition	Cardiac-monitored bed/unit
Monitor	Vitals
	Cardiac monitoring
Diet	?NPO, cardiac diet, low fat, low cholesterol, no caffeine
Fluid	Heplock (flush every shift)
O_2	≥2 L O_2 via NC; keep O_2 saturation >92%
Activity	Bedrest
Dx studies	
Labs	CBC, BMP, calcium, Mg, PO_4, LFT, PT/INR/PTT, TSH, UA, ?troponin q8h
	Troponin q8h × 3, CPK-MB q6h × 4
Radiology and cardiac studies	CXR (PA and lateral), ECG, ?cardiac echo
Special tests	?Myoglobin stat and then q6h (high sensitivity but low specificity)
	?Serum/urine toxicology screen, signal-averaged ECG
Prophylaxis	?
Consults	Cardiology
Nursing	DVT
Avoid	Hypothermia
Management	
• Assess patient, check pulses by Doppler	
• Start CPR	
• Search for probable etiology—6 H's and 6 T's	
Hypoxia	Tension pneumothorax
Hypovolemia	Tamponade
Hypothermia	Thrombosis (PE)

(continued)

TABLE 1–9G: Diagnosis: Pulseless Electric Activity (Continued)	
Hypo- or hyperkalemia	Thrombosis (acute coronary syndrome)
Hydrogen ion (acidosis)	Trauma
	Tablets (drugs)
Wide QRS: possible massive myocardial injury, hyperkalemia, hypoxia, hypothermia	
Wide QRS + slow heart: drug overdose (TCA, β-blockers, calcium channel blockers, digoxin)	
Narrow complex: consider hypovolemia, infection, PE, tamponade	
• Specific causes and their treatments	
PE	
No pulse with CPR, no jugular venous distention (JVD)	
Management: thrombolytic/surgery	
Tension pneumothorax	
No pulse with CPR, JVD, tracheal deviation	
Treatment: needle thoracostomy	
Cardiac tamponade	
No pulse with CPR, JVD, narrow pulse before arrest	
Beck's triad (hypotension, JVD, distant heart sounds)	
Treatment: pericardiocentesis	
Hyperkalemia	
Check ECG (hyperacute T waves)	
Treatment: CaCl → NR → albuterol → insulin + glucose → NR → sodium polystyrene (Kayexalate)	
If no etiology found → consider the following:	
Epinephrine: 1 mg IV q3–5min → NR → atropine, 1 mg IV q3–5min (max: 0.04 mg/kg)	
Source: From American Heart Association.	

TABLE 1–10: Diagnosis: Aortic Dissection	
Disposition	Unit
Monitor	Vitals
	Cardiac monitoring
	Neuromonitoring
Diet	NPO
Fluid	Heplock (flush every shift)
O$_2$	≥2 L O$_2$ via NC; keep O$_2$ saturation >92%
Activity	Strict bedrest with bedside commode
Dx studies	
Labs	CBC, BMP, PT/PTT/INR, troponin q8h, CPK-MB q6h
Radiology and cardiac studies	ECG, CXR (PA and lateral), CT, ?MRI
Special tests	TEE; if not available, then use TTE
	?Aortogram, ?intravascular ultrasonography (can detect dissection even with –Ve TEE)
	?Immunoassay for smooth muscle myosin heavy chain (highly sensitive in first 3 hrs)
Prophylaxis	?
Consults	Cardiothoracic surgery, cardiology
Nursing	Stool guaiac (especially if history of abdominal surgery)
Avoid	Propranolol in patients with bronchoconstriction and sinus bradycardia
Management	See Management: Aortic Dissection
	Sufficient pain management required

(continued)

FIGURE 1–11: Aortic dissection.

De Bakey Type I	Type II	Type III

Stanford	Type A	Type B

TABLE 1–10: Diagnosis: Aortic Dissection (Continued)

Aortic Dissection Classifications

DeBakey classification

Type I: originates in the ascending aorta, propagates at least to the aortic arch and often beyond it distally

Type II: originates in and is confined to the ascending aorta

Type III: originates in the descending aorta and extends distally down the aorta or, rarely, retrogrades into the aortic arch and ascending aorta

Stanford classification

Type A: all dissection involving the ascending aorta, regardless of the site of origin

Type B: all dissection not involving ascending aorta

Source: From Nienaber CA, Eagle KA. Aortic dissection: new frontiers in diagnosis and management: Part I: from etiology to diagnostic strategies. *Circulation* 2003;108:628–635, with permission.

(continued)

TABLE 1–10: Diagnosis: Aortic Dissection (Continued)

Management: Aortic Dissection

Consider surgery if following:

• Acute dissection of ascending aorta

• Acute dissection of descending aorta with:

Signs of impending rupture (persisting pain, hypotension, left-sided hemothorax)

Marfan syndrome

• Chronic dissection if aorta >5–6 cm in diameter or symptoms

Acute BP management

• Propranolol, 0.5–1 mg IV q3–5min, *or* metoprolol, 5 mg IV q5min (keep HR <70)

Then nitroprusside 0.3–10 mg/kg/min to keep SBP 100–120 mm Hg first line

(If nitroprusside is continued for >48 hrs, then check thiocyanate level)

or

• First line: labetalol: 10–20 mg IV bolus followed by 40–80 mg q10min

or

• Second line: trimethaphan: 1–2 mg/min IV infusion

or

• Third line: reserpine: 0.5–2 mg IM q4–8h

or

• Third line: methyldopa: 250–500 mg PO q6h (useful in pregnancy)

Chronic BP management

• Metoprolol, 25–100 mg PO bid *or* atenolol, 50–100 mg PO daily

plus

(continued)

TABLE 1–10: Diagnosis: Aortic Dissection (Continued)
• Clonidine, 0.1–0.3 mg PO/patch daily, *or* hydralazine, 10–50 mg PO qid, *or*
Amlodipine, 2.5–10 mg PO daily, *or* enalapril, 2.5–20 mg PO daily
Pain management
• Morphine, 2–5 mg IV q3–4h
or
• Meperidine, 50–100 mg IV/IM q4h PRN (caution in elderly due to risk of delirium)
GFR 10–50 mL/min, 75% of normal dose at usual intervals
GFR <10 mL/min, 50% of normal dose at usual intervals

2
Endocrinology

TABLE 2–1: Diagnosis: Adrenal Crisis	
Disposition	Unit
Monitor	Vitals
	Cardiac monitoring
	Electrolyte monitoring
Diet	Regular
Fluid	Heplock (flush every shift)
O_2	≥2 L O_2 via NC; keep O_2 saturation >92%
Activity	Bedrest
Dx studies	
Labs	CBC, BMP, calcium, Mg, PO_4, LFT, TSH, T_3 and free T_4, cortisol level
Radiology and cardiac studies	CXR (PA and lateral), ECG, CT of abdomen and head
Special tests	?HIV testing, adrenocorticotropic (ACTH) stimulation test (see following page)
	Renin level, aldosterone level, ACTH level
	Metyrapone tests in suspected ACTH deficiency, 24-hr cortisol level
	PPD in high-risk population
Prophylaxis	DVT
Consults	Endocrinology
Nursing	?
Avoid	K^+ and calcium supplements

(continued)

TABLE 2–1: Diagnosis: Adrenal Crisis (Continued)	
Management	
1. Hypotension with NS or D_5NS (2–3 L): 500 mL/hr to wide open	
2. Dexamethasone sodium phosphate, 4 mg IV, or hydrocortisone, 100 mg IV q6–8h, for first 24 hrs	
(**Note:** Dexamethasone is preferred because it does not interfere with ACTH stimulation test)	
or	
3. Fludrocortisone: 0.1–0.2 mg/day	
4. Steroid dose should be adjusted during stress (infection, pregnancy, surgery)	
ACTH stimulation test	
1. Obtain baseline serum cortisol and ACTH levels.	
2. Administer 0.25 mg of cosyntropin (synthetic ACTH) IV/IM.	
3. Repeat cortisol levels every 30 mins and 6 hrs after ACTH administration (normal >18 mcg/dL).	
4. Normal response is indicated when the cortisol level doubles in response to ACTH stimulation.	
5. In adrenal insufficiency, serum cortisol levels fail to rise after ACTH administration.	
Signs and symptoms	
Nausea/vomiting/dehydration	Anorexia → weight loss
Abdominal pain → "acute abdomen"	Unexplained fever
Hyperpigmentation or vitiligo	Weakness/malaise
Constipation/diarrhea	Syncope
Vitals and lab evaluation	
Hypotension	Unexplained hypoglycemia
Hyponatremia	Hyperkalemia

(continued)

TABLE 2–1: Diagnosis: Adrenal Crisis (Continued)	
Hypercalcemia	Azotemia
Eosinophilia	↑ TSH, and ↓ T_3, T_4
ECG: peaked T waves	CT of abdomen: calcification, enlargement, or hemorrhage of adrenal gland
	CT of head: destruction of pituitary/mass lesion

TABLE 2–2: Diagnosis: Diabetic Ketoacidosis (DKA)	
Disposition	Unit
Monitor	Vitals
	Cardiac monitoring
	Neuro check
	Electrolyte monitoring
Diet	NPO → once stable start American Diabetes Association (ADA) diet, complex carbohydrate diet
Fluid	Caution in patient with CHF
	NS or $1/2$ NS first liter should be given quickly (wide open)
	Then 500 mL–800 L/hr (correct fluid deficit), then start maintenance 150–500 mL/hr
	Change IVF to D_5NS or D_5 $1/2$ NS once the glucose level 250–300 mg/dL
O_2	≥2 L O_2 via NC; keep O_2 saturation >92%
Activity	Strict bedrest with bedside commode
Dx studies	
Labs	CBC with differential, BMP q2h × 2–3, then q4h until electrolyte stabilizes
	Calcium, Mg^+, PO_4, ABG, LFT, troponin q8h × 3, CPK-MB q6h × 4
	β-Hydroxybutyrate (ketone), anion gap
	Fingerstick glucose q1h initially for first 3 hrs, then q2–4h for next 12 hrs
	UA, urine C&S, blood C&S, serum/urine ketone, serum osmolality

(continued)

TABLE 2-2: Diagnosis: Diabetic Ketoacidosis (DKA) (Continued)	
Radiology and cardiac studies	CXR (PA and lateral), ECG
Special tests	Calculate Δ/Δ, HbA1$_C$, amylase, lipase, β-HCG, stool guaiac
Prophylaxis	DVT
Consults	Endocrinology, diabetic education
Nursing	Foley catheter, I/O, urine output, stool guaiac, monitor electrolytes
Avoid	Hypokalemia
Management	See Management: DKA
Note	
• As DKA is being treated, anion gap $\downarrow$, but ketone can $\uparrow$ because the main ketone that is measured is acetoacetate, not β-hydroxybutyrate, and as DKA is being treated, β-hydroxybutyrate converts to acetoacetate.	
Calculation of Replacement of Total Body Water (TBW) Deficit	
1. TBW in hypernatremia = **Male:** $0.5 \times$ wt (kg), **Female:** $0.4 \times$ wt (kg)	
2. TBW in hyponatremia = **Male:** $0.6 \times$ wt (kg), **Female:** = $0.5 \times$ wt (kg)	
3. **Current TBW** = TBW $\times$ $(140/P_{Na^+})$	
4. **TBW deficit** = TBW $-$ current TBW	
5. **X** = replacement fluid Na$^+$ (mEq)/154	
6. **Replacement volume (L)** = TBW deficit $\times [1/(1 - X)]$	
Example	
1. A 70-kg male with P_{Na^+} of 160 mEq/L	
2. TBW = $(0.5 \times 70$ kg$) = 35$ L	
3. Current TBW = $[35 \times (140/160)] = 30.6$ L	

(continued)

TABLE 2–2: Diagnosis: Diabetic Ketoacidosis (DKA) (Continued)

4. TBW deficit = $(35 - 30.6) = 4.4$ L

5. $X = 75$ (mEq/L)/154 = 0.49

6. Replacement volume (L) = 4.4 L $\times [1/(1 - 0.49)] = 8.6$ L (replace this deficit in 48–72 hrs)

Note

- Correct sodium for hyperglycemia; for each 100 mg/dL ↑ of blood sugar above 200 mg/dL, Na^+ can ↓ 1.6 mEq

- Replacement: Give one-half in first 24 hrs and next half in next 48 hrs

- Isotonic fluid (NS) should be used initially when correcting TBW deficit and should be corrected slowly over 48–72 hrs

- The serum sodium should fall by no more than 0.5 mEq/L/hr (12 mEq/day)

- Na^+ concentration in IV fluids: NS = 154 mEq/L, $1/2$ NS = 75 mEq/L

Management: DKA

1. If K^+ is <3.3 → replace K^+ before giving insulin (ADA recommendation)

2. Initially: regular insulin, 0.1–0.2 U/kg IV followed by infusion of 0.1 U/kg/hr IV

   Note: Infusion: 100 U in 500 mL NS (infusion rate of 50 mL/hr gives 10 U/hr)

   An appropriate response to insulin treatment is ↓ blood glucose of 50–75 mg/dL/hr

3. ↓ Insulin infusion rate to 2–3 U/hr when glucose level ↓ to 250–300

4. Stop insulin infusion when anion gap normalizes (10–15) and HCO_3 is close to normal; give SQ insulin before stopping infusion (IV insulin half-life is only a few minutes)

(continued)

TABLE 2–2: Diagnosis: Diabetic Ketoacidosis (DKA) (Continued)
5. **K^+:** Potassium depletion should be expected with insulin treatment; if K^+ <4 → replace with IV boluses → add 20–40 mEq KCl to each liter of IVF → change to K^+ phosphate to prevent chloride overload (monitor K^+ q2h)
Vigorously replace K^+
Peripheral IV: KCl, 10 mEq/hr
Central line: 20 mEq/hr or nasogastric (NG) tube
If PO tolerated, 40–80 mEq
If concurrent K^+ and PO_4 depletion → consider potassium phosphate, 20–40 mEq
6. **PO_4:** If PO_4 <1 mEq/L (ADA recommendation) → give phosphorus, 2.5–5 mg/kg in 500 mL over 6 hrs
7. **Mg:** Replacement is required only if severe hypomagnesemia or refractory hypokalemia
Patients with ventricular arrhythmia → treat with magnesium sulfate, 2.5–5 g IV
8. **HCO_3:** not required unless patient's pH ≤7 (ADA recommendation); treatment: add 50–100 mEq HCO_3 to each liter
9. Headache: acetaminophen (Tylenol), 325–650 mg PO q4–6h
10. Treat underlying etiology (e.g., infection, MI, noncompliance)

Sample of Electrolyte Monitoring Table						
Time	**Blood sugar**	**Na/K/ PO_4**	**Anion gap**	**I/O**	**Current treatment**	**Plan**

TABLE 2–3: Diagnosis: Nonketotic Hyperosmolar Syndrome (NKHS)	
Disposition	Unit
Monitor	Vitals
	Cardiac monitoring
	Electrolyte monitor
Diet	NPO → once stable start ADA diet
Fluid	NS, 1–2 L over 1 hr (caution in patient with CHF) → NS, 500 mL/hr until fluid deficit is corrected → start maintenance $1/2$ NS at 150–125 mL/hr → IVF should be changed to D_5NS or D_5 $1/2$ NS when glucose level reaches 250–300 mg/dL
O_2	≥2 L O_2 via NC; keep O_2 saturation >92%
Activity	Strict bedrest with bedside commode
Dx studies	
Labs	CBC with differential, BMP q2h × 2–3, then q4h until electrolyte stabilizes
	Calcium, LFT, Mg^+, PO_4, ABG, troponin
	Anion gap, β-hydroxybutyrate (ketone)
	Fingerstick glucose q1h initially for first 3 hrs, then q2–4h for next 12 hrs
	UA, urine and blood C&S, serum/urine ketones, serum osmolality
Radiology and cardiac studies	CXR (PA and lateral), ECG
Special tests	Calculate Δ/Δ, $HbA1_C$, stool guaiac, β-HCG, amylase, lipase
Prophylaxis	DVT
Consults	Endocrinology, diabetic education

(continued)

TABLE 2–3: Diagnosis: Nonketotic Hyperosmolar Syndrome (NKHS) (Continued)	
Nursing	Foley, I/O, urine output hourly (maintain 50 mL/hr)
Avoid	Hypokalemia
Management	See Management: Nonketotic Hyperosmolar Syndrome

Calculation of Replacement of Total Body Water (TBW) Deficit

1. TBW in hypernatremia = **Male:** $0.5 \times$ wt (kg), **Female:** $0.4 \times$ wt (kg)

2. **Current TBW** = TBW $\times (140/P_{Na^+})$

3. **TBW deficit** = TBW − current TBW

4. **X** = Replacement fluid Na^+ (mEq)/154

5. **Replacement volume (L)** = TBW deficit $\times [1/(1 - X)]$

Example

1. A 70-kg male with P_{Na^+} of 160 mEq/L

2. TBW = $(0.5 \times 70$ kg$) = 35$ L

3. Current TBW = $[35 \times (140/160)] = 30.6$ L

4. TBW deficit = $(35 - 30.6) = 4.4$ L

5. X = 75 (mEq/L)/154 = 0.49

6. Replacement volume (L) = 4.4 L $\times [1/(1 - 0.49)] = 8.6$ L (replace deficit in 48–72 hrs)

Note

- Replacement: Give one-half in first 24 hrs and next half in next 48 hrs.

- Isotonic fluid (NS) should be used initially when correcting TBW deficit and should be corrected slowly over 48–72 hrs.

- The serum sodium should fall by no more than 0.5 mEq/L/hr (12 mEq/day).

(continued)

TABLE 2–3: Diagnosis: Nonketotic Hyperosmolar Syndrome (NKHS) (Continued)

• Na^+ concentration in IV fluids: NS = 154 mEq/L, 1/2 NS = 75 mEq/L.

Management: Nonketotic Hyperosmolar Syndrome

1. Fluid replacement and electrolyte replacement essential

   Note: If K^+ <3.3 → replace K^+ before giving insulin

2. Calculate serum osmolarity: $(2 \times Na^+) + (BUN/2.8) + (glucose/18)$

3. NS → 1–1.5 L/hr initially, then change to 1/2 NS at 500 mL/hr

4. Regular insulin, 0.1–0.2 U, should be given initially in severe hyperglycemia (>600) then

   Infusion: 0.05–0.1 U/kg/hr (50 U of regular insulin in 500 mL of NS at 50 mL/hr gives 5 U/hr)

5. When glucose reaches 250–300 mg/dL → ↓ infusion rate to 1–2 U/hr and change IVF to D_5 1/2 NS

6. After stopping infusion → place patient on sliding scale and regular insulin SQ

7. **K^+:** Potassium depletion should be expected with insulin treatment; if K^+ <4 → replace with IV boluses → add 20–40 mEq KCl to each liter of IVF → change to K^+ phosphate to prevent chloride overload (monitor K^+ q2h)

   Vigorously replace K^+

   Peripheral IV: KCl, 10 mEq/hr

   Central line: 20 mEq/hr or NG tube

   If PO tolerated, 40–80 mEq

   If concurrent K^+ and PO_4 depletion → consider potassium phosphate, 20–40 mEq

8. **PO_4:** If PO_4 <1 mEq/L → phosphorus, 2.5–5 mg/kg in 500 mL over 6 hrs

(continued)

TABLE 2–3: Diagnosis: Nonketotic Hyperosmolar Syndrome (NKHS) (Continued)
9. **Mg:** Replacement is required only if severe hypomagnesemia or refractory hypokalemia
Patients with ventricular arrhythmia → treat with magnesium sulfate, 2.5–5 g IV
10. **HCO_3:** not required unless patient's pH ≤7; treatment: add 50–100 mEq HCO_3 to each liter
11. Headache: Tylenol, 325–650 mg PO q4–6h
12. Treat underlying etiology (e.g., infection, MI, noncompliance)

			Sample of Electrolyte Monitoring Table			
Time	Blood sugar	Na/K/ PO_4	Anion gap	I/O	Current treatment	Plan

TABLE 2–4: Diagnosis: Thyroid Storm (Thyrotoxicosis)	
Disposition	Unit
Monitor	Vitals
	Cardiac monitoring
	Electrolyte monitoring
Diet	NPO
Fluid	Heplock (flush every shift)
O_2	≥ 2 L O_2 via NC; keep O_2 saturation >92%
Activity	Bedrest
Dx studies	
Labs	Stat total T_4 (primary turnaround), BMP, calcium, Mg, PO_4, TSH, free T_4, total T_3
	CBC with differential, β-HCG in females, blood and urine C&S, CPK (r/o rhabdomyolysis), LFT
Radiology studies	CXR (PA and lateral), ECG, ?thyroid scan, ?US of thyroid
Special tests	?Serum and urine toxicology screen, ?ETOH level, ?troponin, ?radioiodine uptake
	?Nuclear thyroid scintigraphy ^{123}I [cannot perform nuclear scan after saturated solution of potassium iodide (SSKI)]
Prophylaxis	DVT
Consults	Endocrinology
Nursing	?
Avoid	ASA (displaces T_4 from thyroid-binding globulin, thus raising T_4 level)
	β-Blocker in bronchoconstriction
	Anticoagulation activity may be ↑ by propylthiouracil (PTU)
Management	See Management: Thyroid Storm

(continued)

TABLE 2–4: Diagnosis: Thyroid Storm (Thyrotoxicosis) (Continued)			
Diagnostic Criteria for Thyroid Storm			
Signs and symptoms	**Score**	**Signs and symptoms**	**Score**
Tachycardia		CNS	
99–109	5	Mild agitation	10
110–119	10	Moderate delirium	20
120–129	15	Moderate psychosis	20
130–139	20	Extreme lethargy	20
>140	25	Severe seizure/coma	30
Temperature		CHF	
99–99.9	5	Mild pedal edema	5
100–100.9	10	Moderate bibasilar rales	10
101–101.9	15	Severe pulmonary edema	15
102–102.9	20	Atrial fibrillation	10
103–103.9	25	Precipitant history	
>104	30	Negative	0
GI		Positive	10
Moderate nausea/ vomiting/diarrhea, abdominal pain	10		
Severe unexplained jaundice	20		
<25, storm is unlikely; 25–44 supports the diagnosis of storm, ≥45 highly suggestive of storm.			
Source: From Burch HB, Wartofsky L. Life-threatening thyrotoxicosis: thyroid storm. *Endocrinol Metab Clin North Am* 1993;22:263, with permission.			

(continued)

TABLE 2–4: Diagnosis: Thyroid Storm (Thyrotoxicosis) (Continued)
Management: Thyroid Storm
• Adjust dosing of PTU and methimazole in pregnancy ($\downarrow$ dose)
• PTU: 300–600 mg PO/NG bolus, then 150–300 mg PO/NG q6h
(Preferred in elderly, cardiac disease, and pregnant and lactating females) *or*
Methimazole (Tapazole): 80–100 mg PO/PR/NG bolus, then 30 mg q8h
• Saturated solution of potassium iodide: 5 drops PO q6–8h × 24–72 hrs, *or*
Sodium iodine: 250 mg IV q6h, *or*
Lugol's solution: 10 drops added to IVF q8h
• Propranolol: 80–120 mg PO q4–6h *or* 1 mg/min for 2–10 mins (blocks T_4 and T_3) *or*
Esmolol: 5g in 500 mL D_5W, loading dose of 500 mcg/kg over 1 min, then 50–200 mcg/kg/min
• Dexamethasone: 2 mg IV q6–8h, *or* hydrocortisone, 100 mg IV q6–8h
• Tylenol: 325–650 mg PO q6h PRN for fever
• CHF and atrial fibrillation: Manage with digoxin
• [131]Iodine and surgery reserved until patient is euthyroid
Note: Administer PTU or methimazole 1 hr before giving iodide to prevent oxidation of iodide to iodine.

TABLE 2–5: Diagnosis: Myxedema Coma	
Disposition	Unit
Monitor	Vitals (hypothermia)
	Cardiac monitoring
	Electrolyte monitoring (hyponatremia, hypoglycemia)
Diet	High bulk diet (to prevent constipation)
Fluid	IV hydration essential (caution in patient with CHF)
O₂	≥2 L O_2 via NC; keep O_2 saturation >92%; respiratory support essential
Activity	Bedrest
Dx studies	
Labs	CBC with differential, BMP, calcium, Mg, PO_4 level, TSH, free T_4, total T_3, T_4, LFT
	β-HCG in females, ABG, CPK, blood and urine C&S, lipid profile
	Cortisol level before and after cosyntropin (Cortrosyn) administration (r/o adrenal insufficiency)
Radiology studies	CXR (PA and lateral), ECG, ?head CT (r/o CVA)
Special tests	Troponin q8h × 3, CPK-MB q6h × 3, ?radioiodine uptake
Prophylaxis	DVT
Consults	Endocrinology
Nursing	?
Avoid	β-Blocker, antihypertensives, narcotics can ↑ T_4, sedatives

(continued)

TABLE 2–5: Diagnosis: Myxedema Coma (Continued)
Management
• Prevent heat loss: Cover the patient but avoid external rewarming to prevent vascular collapse
• Respiratory support
• Thyroxine: 200–400 mcg IV followed by 50–100 mcg daily
• Triiodothyronine: 5–20 mcg IV followed by 2.5–10 mcg IV q8h
• Hydrocortisone: 100 mg IV q8h; give before thyroid replacement
Note: Sudden change in metabolic rate after treatment may precipitate ACS in these patients; consider anticoagulation in patients at high risk or in patients with prior atrial fibrillation.

TABLE 2–6: Diagnosis: Hyperparathyroidism and Severe Hypercalcemia	
Disposition	Medical floor/unit
Monitor	Vitals
	Cardiac monitoring
	Electrolyte monitoring
Diet	Limit calcium to 1,200–1,500 mg/day and vitamin D to 400 IU/day
Fluid	IVF hydration essential before diuresis
O₂	PRN
Activity	As tolerated
Dx studies	
Labs	CBC, BMP, Mg, PO₄, ionized calcium, albumin, LFT, parathyroid hormone (PTH)
Radiology and cardiac studies	ECG, CXR (PA and lateral)
	?CT of neck with and without contrast, immunoassay for intact PTH
	?Sestamibi scan for neck, ?thallium technetium scan of neck (to localize lesion)
Special tests	Amylase, lipase, PTH, iPTH assay
	24-hr urine calcium, ?calcitriol
	?PTH-like protein (associated with solid malignancy), PTHrP
Prophylaxis	?
Consults	Endocrinology, ?nephrology
Avoid	Thiazide diuretic, calcium-containing products
Management	See Management: Hyperparathyroidism and Hypercalcemia

(continued)

TABLE 2–6: Diagnosis: Hyperparathyroidism and Severe Hypercalcemia (Continued)	
Hyperparathyroidism	
Signs and symptoms	
Hypercalcemia	Nephrolithiasis
Anemia	Bone disease
Hypophosphatemia	Proximal/distal renal tubular acidosis
Hypomagnesemia	↑ Calcitriol production
Hyperuricemia	Muscle weakness
Weakness and fatigue	↑ Gastrin production → peptic ulcer
Constipation	Nephrogenic diabetes insipidus
Pancreatitis	Corneal calcium deposition
Shortening of Q-T interval	CNS dysfunction

PTH inhibits proximal tubular bicarbonate reabsorption → mild metabolic acidosis.

Management: Hyperparathyroidism and Severe Hypercalcemia

- Treat hypercalcemia (also see Chapter 6)

- IVF: NS at 200–300 mL/hr → adjust to maintain the urinary output to 100–150 mL/hr followed by furosemide (Lasix) diuretics

- Zoledronic acid: 4 mg IV over 15 mins

- Calcitonin: 4 IU/kg q12h if NS and Lasix not effective

- Pamidronate: 60–90 mg IV over 4 hr q24h (if serum calcium >3.5 mg/dL)

- Etidronate, 7.5 mg/kg/24 hr IV daily × 3 days, or alendronate, 5–10 mg PO qd or 70 mg PO weekly

- Prednisone: 20 mg PO bid–tid

(continued)

TABLE 2–6: Diagnosis: Hyperparathyroidism and Severe Hypercalcemia (Continued)
• Gallium nitrate: 200 mg IV continuous infusion for 5 days (side effect: nephrotoxicity), not commonly used
• Dialysis
• Treat underlying etiology

3
Gastroenterology

TABLE 3–1: Diagnosis: Cholecystitis	
Disposition	Surgical/medical floor
Monitor	Vitals
Diet	NPO
Fluid	MIVF
O$_2$	PRN
Activity	Bedrest
Dx studies	
Labs	CBC with differential, BMP, Mg, LFT, lipid profile, amylase, lipase, γ-glutamyl transpeptidase (GGTP)
	Blood C&S, PT/PTT/INR, UA
Radiology and cardiac studies	If RUQ US negative→ HIDA scan (cholescintigraphy), CXR, ECG
Special tests	?Morphine cholescintigraphy, ?MR cholangiography, ?CT of abdomen
	?Endoscopic retrograde cholangio-pancreatography (ERCP) (if bile duct obstruction from stone), ?acute abdominal x-ray series
Prophylaxis	DVT
Consults	Surgery, ?GI
Nursing	?
Avoid	?

(continued)

TABLE 3–1: Diagnosis: Cholecystitis (Continued)
Management
Supportive management
• Treat N/V with PRN medications
• Pain management: See Chapter 12 [commonly used: morphine, hydromorphone (Dilaudid)]
Ampicillin/sulbactam (Unasyn): 3 g q6h IV first line
Piperacillin/tazobactam (Zosyn): 3.375 g q6h IV first line
Ampicillin plus gentamicin (adjust for renal dose) first line (see dosing below)
Ticarcillin/clavulanate (Timentin): 3.1 g q6h IV first line
Third-generation cephalosporin plus metronidazole (500 mg PO qid or 15 mg/kg IV q12h) second line
Aztreonam, 2 g IV q8h, plus metronidazole (500 mg PO qid or 15 mg/kg IV q12h) second line
Ciprofloxacin, 400 mg IV q12h, plus metronidazole (500 mg PO qid or 15 mg/kg IV q12h) second line
Meropenem second line (see dosing on following page)
Levofloxacin third line (see dosing on following page)
• Ampicillin, 2 g IV q6h, plus gentamicin (see dosing below) ± metronidazole, 500 mg IV/PO q8h
• Gentamicin: 2–2.5 mg/kg q8h (adjust dosing in renal impairment)
• CrCl ≥60 mL/min: Administer q8h
• CrCl 40–60 mL/min: Administer q12h
• CrCl 20–40 mL/min: Administer q24h
• CrCl 10–20 mL/min: Administer q48h
• CrCl <10 mL/min: Administer q72h

(continued)

TABLE 3–1: Diagnosis: Cholecystitis (Continued)
• Meropenem: 1g IV q8h (adjust dosing in renal impairment)
• CrCl 26–50 mL/min: Administer 1 g q12h
• CrCl 10–25 mL/min: Administer 500 mg q12h
• CrCl <10 mL/min: Administer 500 mg q24h
• Levofloxacin: 500 mg IV q24h (adjust dosing in renal impairment)
• CrCl 20–49 mL/min: 250 mg q24h
• CrCl 10–19 mL/min: 250 mg q48h

TABLE 3–2: Diagnosis: Cholangitis	
Disposition	Unit
Monitor	Vitals, temperature
Diet	NPO
Fluid	MIVF
O$_2$	PRN
Activity	Bedrest
Dx studies	
Labs	CBC with differential, BMP, LFT, blood C&S, amylase, lipase, GGTP
	Blood C&S, PT/PTT/INR, UA
Radiology and cardiac studies	RUQ US, CT of abdomen, ?acute abdominal x-ray series, CXR, ECG
Special tests	?ERCP (if bile duct obstruction from stone)
Prophylaxis	DVT
Consults	GI, surgery, ?ID
Nursing	?
Avoid	Aminoglycoside in cirrhosis
Management	
Supportive management	
• Treat N/V with PRN medications	
• Pain management: See Chapter 12 (commonly used medications: morphine, Dilaudid)	
Piperacillin/tazobactam (Zosyn): 3.375 g q6h IV first line	
Unasyn: 3 g q6h IV first line	
Ampicillin plus gentamicin (adjust for renal dose) first line (see dosing on following page)	

(continued)

TABLE 3–2: Diagnosis: Cholangitis (Continued)

Timentin: 3.1 g q6h IV first line

Third-generation cephalosporin plus metronidazole (500 mg PO qid or 15 mg/kg IV q12h) second line

Aztreonam, 2 g IV q8h, plus metronidazole (500 mg PO qid or 15 mg/kg IV q12h) second line

Ciprofloxacin, 400 mg IV q12h, plus metronidazole (500 mg PO qid or 15 mg/kg IV q12h) second line

Meropenem second line (see dosing below)

Levofloxacin third line (see dosing below)

• Ampicillin, 2 g IV q6h, plus gentamicin (see dosing below) ± metronidazole, 500 mg IV/PO q8h

• Gentamicin: 2–2.5 mg/kg q8h (adjust dosing in renal impairment)

  • CrCl ≥60 mL/min: Administer q8h

  • CrCl 40–60 mL/min: Administer q12h

  • CrCl 20–40 mL/min: Administer q24h

  • CrCl 10–20 mL/min: Administer q48h

  • CrCl <10 mL/min: Administer q72h

• Meropenem: 1g IV q8h (adjust dosing in renal impairment)

  • CrCl 26–50 mL/min: Administer 1 g q12h

  • CrCl 10–25 mL/min: Administer 500 mg q12h

  • CrCl <10 mL/min: Administer 500 mg q24h

• Levofloxacin: 500 mg IV q24h (adjust dosing in renal impairment)

  • CrCl 20–49 mL/min: 250 mg q24h

  • CrCl 10–19 mL/min: 250 mg q48h

TABLE 3–3: Diagnosis: Crohn's Disease	
Disposition	Medical floor
Monitor	Vitals
Diet	NPO except ice chips and medications for 48 hrs → start elemental or low residue diet
Fluid	MIVF; hydration essential
O₂	PRN
Activity	Bedrest
Dx studies	
Labs	CBC, BMP, calcium, Mg, ionized calcium, LFT, UA, blood C&S × 2
	Stool leukocyte and C&S, stool Wright's stain, stool ova and parasite
Radiology and cardiac studies	Abdóminal x-ray series, CXR, CT of abdomen, ?colonoscopy
Special tests	?CRP, ?ESR, ?p-ANCA (commonly associated with ulcerative colitis), ?anti-*Saccharomyces cerevisiae* antibodies (commonly associated with Crohn's disease), ?*Clostridium difficile* toxin A and B
Prophylaxis	DVT
Consults	GI
Nursing	I/O, stool guaiac
Avoid	Dairy products
Management	
• Multivitamin: 1 tablet PO daily or 1 ampule IV daily	
• Folic acid: 1 mg PO daily	

(continued)

TABLE 3–3: Diagnosis: Crohn's Disease (Continued)

- If vitamin B_{12} deficiency → vitamin B_{12} 100 mcg IM × 5 days, then 100 mcg IM every mo

- Methylprednisolone (Solu-Medrol), 10–20 mg IV q6h, *or* prednisone, 40–60 mg PO daily

- Mesalamine (Asacol): 400–800 mg PO tid–qid *or*

  Mesalamine (Pentasa): 250 mg PO qid *or*

  Sulfasalazine: 0.5–1g PO q6h *or*

  Olsalazine: 500 mg PO bid *or*

  Mesalamine: 1 g PO q6h

- Etanercept (Infliximab): 5 mg/kg IV over 2 hrs

- ?Metronidazole: 250–500 mg PO q6h

TABLE 3–4: Diagnosis: Hepatic Encephalopathy	
Disposition	Unit
Monitor	Vitals
	?Cardiac monitoring
	Electrolyte monitoring
	Neuromonitoring: neuro check q2–4h
Diet	NPO initially, then protein restriction diet (protein intake of 40–70 g/day)
Fluid	MIVF
O_2	≥2 L O_2 via NC; keep O_2 saturation >92%
Activity	Bedrest
Dx studies	
Labs	Ammonia, CBC with differential, BMP, calcium, Mg, PO_4, PT/PTT/INR, UA, ABG, LDH
	LFT, GGTP, urine C&S and blood C&S × 2
	ABG, serum toxicology screen, acetaminophen (Tylenol), ASA level, ESR
	Hepatitis panel (HepBsAg, HepB IgM, HepB IgG, Hep C IgG, Hep C IgM)
Radiology and cardiac studies	CXR, ECG, US of abdomen, CT of abdomen
Special tests	CRP, ceruloplasmin, ?DIC panel, iron studies (hemochromatosis)
	Copper and ceruloplasmin, urine copper (Wilson's disease)
	α_1-Antitrypsin globulin on SPEP (α_1-antitrypsin deficiency)

(continued)

TABLE 3–4: Diagnosis: Hepatic Encephalopathy (Continued)	
	Antimitochondrial antibody (primary biliary cirrhosis)
	p-ANCA (primary sclerosing cholangitis)
Prophylaxis	GI prophylaxis
Consults	GI, transplant
Nursing	Stool guaiac, Foley catheter, seizure precaution, I/O, neuro check
Avoid	Heparin, warfarin (Coumadin), narcotics, Tylenol, NSAIDs, sedatives, protein, benzodiazepines, herbal medications, diphenoxylate hydrochloride and atropine (Lomotil)
Management	
• If INR elevated → vitamin K, 10 mg SQ daily	
If bleeding → consider FFP and PRBC transfusion	
• Sorbitol: 70% solution 30–60 g PO	
• Lactulose: 30–50 mL PO q1h, then 15–40 mL PO bid–tid (titrate to achieve two to three soft stools/day) *or*	
Lactulose enema: 300–700 mL tap water; give 200–250 mL bid–qid via rectal tube	
• Lactobacillus SF 68, ornithine-aspartate, benzoate	
• Fermentable fibers, sodium benzoate 5 g bid	
• Neomycin: 1–2 g PO q6h (max: 8–12 g/day, associated with ototoxicity and nephrotoxicity) *or*	
Metronidazole, 250 mg PO q6h, *or* paromomycin *or* rifaximin	
• Thiamine: 100 mg IV/PO daily	
• Folic acid: 1 mg IV/PO daily	
• Multivitamin: 1 ampule IV daily or 1 tablet PO daily	

(continued)

TABLE 3–4: Diagnosis: Hepatic Encephalopathy (Continued)

- Flumazenil: 0.2 mg (2 mL) IV every min until dose of 3 mg reached; if patient responds partially, then give the same dose up to total of 5 mg (may help reverse hepatic encephalopathy despite benzodiazepine use)

- ?Modified amino acid solution ("COMA" solution), ?L-dopa, ?bromocriptine

- ?Zinc

- Melatonin for sleep disturbance

- Consider transplantation if above modalities fail

Stages of Encephalopathy

I	II	III	IV
Change in mental status	Lethargy and confusion	Stupor	Coma

Etiology of Hepatic Encephalopathy in Patients with Cirrhosis

Medications

  Benzodiazepines

  ETOH

  Narcotics

First-degree hepatocellular carcinoma

↑ **Ammonia production**

  ↑ Protein intake

  GI bleeding

  Infection

  Hypokalemia

  Constipation

  Metabolic alkalosis

(continued)

TABLE 3–4: Diagnosis: Hepatic Encephalopathy (Continued)
Dehydration
Vomiting
Diarrhea
Hemorrhage
Diuretics
Vascular occlusion
Portal venous thrombosis
Hepatic venous thrombosis
Portosystemic shunting
Radiographic shunt
Surgically placed shunt
Spontaneous shunt

TABLE 3–5: Diagnosis: Intestinal Obstruction	
Disposition	Medical/surgical floor, ?monitor floor
Monitor	Vitals
	Electrolyte monitoring
Diet	NPO
Fluid	MIVF
O$_2$	PRN
Activity	Bedrest
Dx studies	
Labs	CBC, BMP, calcium, Mg, PO$_4$, LFT, PT/ PTT/INR, amylase, lipase, UA, urine C&S
	Blood C&S, lactic acid, β-HCG if female
Radiology and cardiac studies	Abdominal x-ray, CT of abdomen, ?upper GI and small bowel series
	?Gastrografin or barium enema (contraindicated if perforation)
	CXR (PA and lateral), pelvic and abdominal US
Special tests	?Flexible colonoscopy
Prophylaxis	DVT
Consults	Surgery
Nursing	NG tube with suction, stool guaiac
Avoid	Narcotics
Management	Treat underlying cause

(continued)

TABLE 3–5: Diagnosis: Intestinal Obstruction (Continued)		
Etiology of Intestinal Obstruction		
Hernia	Gallstones	Adhesion in history of previous surgery
Tumor	Intussusception	Radiation-induced enteritis
Volvulus	Impacted stool	Granulomatous processes (abnormal tissue growth)
Lead poisoning	Ascaris	Foreign body (bezoar)
Paralytic ileus		
Abdominal injury		Medications (mainly narcotics)
Metabolic disturbances (K^+)		Intraperitoneal infection
Complication of abdominal surgery		Mesenteric ischemia

TABLE 3–6: Diagnosis: Pancreatitis (Acute)	
Disposition	Unit
Monitor	Vitals
	Cardiac monitoring if hemodynamically unstable
Diet	NPO, ?TPN until amylase and lipase normalizes
Fluid	Replace deficit with NS, then MIVF
O_2	PRN
Activity	Bedrest and advance as tolerated slowly (usually after pain is relieved second to fourth day)
Dx studies	
Labs	CBC with differential, BMP, Mg, calcium, PO_4, amylase, lipase, lipid panel, LDH, UA
	PT/PTT/INR, LFT, blood C&S
Radiology and cardiac studies	US of RUQ, CT of abdomen with contrast (r/o pseudocyst/AAA), ?CXR, ?ERCP
Special tests	ECG, ?HepBsAg, hepatitis A
	?Blood C&S, ?stool guaiac, ?serum/urine toxicology, ?UA, urine C&S
	?Secretin stimulation test, ?para-amino-benzoic acid test
Prophylaxis	DVT
Consults	?GI, ?surgery
Nursing	I/O, urine output, NG tube if nausea or vomiting, fingerstick glucose qid, Foley catheter

(continued)

TABLE 3–6: Diagnosis: Pancreatitis (Acute) (Continued)		
Avoid	See medications listed below	
Management	See Management: Pancreatitis	
Etiologies of Pancreatitis		
Gallstones	ETOH	Hyperlipidemia (I, IV, V)
Hypercalcemia	Trauma	Atheroembolism
Pancreatic cancer	Duodenal stricture/ obstruction	Post-ERCP
Ampullary stenosis	Scorpion venom	Pregnancy
Renal transplant	α_1-Antitrypsin deficiency	Choledochocele
Vasculitis	Medications (see below)	Infections (see below)
Medications associated with pancreatitis		
ACE inhibitor	Thiazides	Furosemide
5-ASA	Azathioprine	Didanosine
Estrogen	Pentamidine	L-asparaginase
Metronidazole	Sulindac	Salicylates (ASA)
Stibogluconate	Protease inhibitor	Sulfasalazine
Tetracycline	6-Mercaptopurine	Valproic acid

(continued)

TABLE 3–6: Diagnosis: Pancreatitis (Acute) (Continued)		
Infections associated with pancreatitis		
Ascaris	*Aspergillus*	CMV/EBV
Coxsackie	*Cryptosporidium*	Hepatitis A and B
HIV	HSV	*Legionella*
Leptospira	*Mycoplasma*	Mumps/rubella
Salmonella	*Toxoplasma*	Varicella zoster
Ranson's Criteria		
0 Hrs (GA LAW)	**48 Hrs (C HOBBS)**	
Give one point for each category		
• Age >55 yrs	• HCT ↓ by ≥10%	
• WBC >16,000/μL	• BUN ↑ by ≥5 mg/dL (1.8 mmol/L)	
• Glucose >200 mg/dL (11.1 mmol/L)	• Calcium <8 mEq/L (2 mmol/L)	
• LDH >350 IU/L	• PaO_2 <60 mm Hg	
• AST >250 IU/L	• Base deficit >4 mEq/L	
• ALT >80 IU/L	• Fluid sequestration >6 L	
Prognosis		
Total score	**Mortality**	
≤2	<5%	
3–4	15–20%	
5–6	40%	
≥7	>99%	

(continued)

TABLE 3–6: Diagnosis: Pancreatitis (Acute) (Continued)
Management: Acute Pancreatitis
• Pain management
Morphine: 2–5 mg IV q3–4h
or
Meperidine: 50–100 mg IV/IM q3–4h PRN (caution in elderly due to risk of delirium)
GFR 10–50 mL/min: 75% of normal dose at normal intervals
GFR <10 mL/min: 50% of normal dose at usual intervals
or
Fentanyl: 50–100 mcg/dose q1–2h as needed
Other: Tylenol #3, acetaminophen and hydrocodone (Vicodin)
• Ranitidine, 50 mg IV q6–8h/famotidine, 20 mg IV q12h (to reduce acid release from stomach) *or*
Famotidine, 20 mg IV q12h
• Pancreatic enzyme supplement [pancrelipase (Pancrease MT, Creon)]
• If there is necrotizing pancreatitis (involving more than 30% of the pancreas) → initiate antimicrobial therapy with imipenem/cilastatin (Primaxin), 0.5–1 g IV q6h; continue for at least 7 days
• If infected pseudocyst or abscess:
Timentin: 3.1 g IV or
Unasyn: 3 g IV q6h or
Primaxin: 0.5–1 g IV q6h
• Consider CT-guided aspiration if no improvement with antibiotic therapy

TABLE 3–7: Diagnosis: Peritonitis			
Disposition	Medical floor		
Monitor	Vitals		
	Electrolyte monitoring		
Diet	NPO		
Fluid	MIVF		
O$_2$	PRN		
Activity	Bedrest		
Dx studies			
Labs	CBC with differential, BMP, Mg, LFT, PT/PTT/INR, lactic acid, amylase, lipase		
	UA, urine R&M, urine C&S, ammonia, blood C&S × 2		
Radiology and cardiac studies	Abdominal x-ray (upright and lateral decubitus), CXR (PA and lateral), ECG		
	CT of abdomen, US of abdomen		
Special tests	?GGTP, paracentesis tubes		
	Tube 1	**Tube 2**	**Tube 3**
	Cell count and differential	Glucose	Gram stain
		Protein	Aerobic and anaerobic C&S
		Albumin	
		LDH	
		TG	Fungal C&S
		Amylase	AFB
		Bilirubin	
		Specific gravity	
Prophylaxis	?		

(continued)

TABLE 3–7: Diagnosis: Peritonitis (Continued)	
Consults	Surgery, ?ID
Nursing	Stool guaiac, ?NG tube
Avoid	?

Management: Peritonitis (Bacterial)

Mild–moderate (2° from appendicitis, diverticulitis, etc.)

• Ceftriaxone, 1–2 g IV q24h, plus metronidazole, 1 g IV q24h first line

• Moxifloxacin, 400 mg IV q24h, or Unasyn, 1.5 g q6h, or ceftizoxime, 2 g IV q8h, or cefoxitin, 2 g IV q6h second line

Severe peritonitis (2° from appendicitis, diverticulitis, etc.)

• Meropenem: 1 g IV q8h first line

• Piperacillin/tazobactam: 4.5 g IV q8h first line

• Ertapenem: 1 g IV q24h first line

• Imipenem: 500 mg IV q6h first line

Spontaneous bacterial peritonitis

• Ceftriaxone: 1 g IV q24h first line

• Ciprofloxacin: 400 mg IV or 500 mg PO q12h first line

• Gatifloxacin: 400 mg IV/PO q24h first line

• Levofloxacin: 500 mg IV/PO q24h first line

• Moxifloxacin: 400 mg IV/PO q24h first line

• Aztreonam: 2 g IV q8h second line

TABLE 3–8: Diagnosis: Ulcerative Colitis	
Disposition	Medical floor
Monitor	Vitals
Diet	NPO except ice chips and medications for 48 hrs → start elemental or low-residue diet
Fluid	Hydration essential
O$_2$	PRN
Activity	Bedrest
Dx studies	
Labs	CBC, BMP, calcium, LFT, Mg, ionized calcium, blood C&S × 2, UA
	Stool leukocyte and C&S, stool Wright's stain, stool ova and parasite
Radiology and cardiac studies	Abdominal x-ray series, CXR, colonoscopy, CT of abdomen
Special tests	?CRP, ?ESR, ?p-ANCA (commonly associated with ulcerative colitis), ?anti-*Saccharomyces cerevisiae* antibodies (commonly associated with Crohn's disease)
	?*C. difficile* toxin A and B
Prophylaxis	DVT
Consults	GI
Nursing	I/O, stool guaiac
Avoid	Dairy products
Management	
• Multivitamin: 1 tablet PO daily or 1 ampule IV daily	
• Folic acid: 1 mg PO daily	

(continued)

TABLE 3–8: Diagnosis: Ulcerative Colitis (Continued)

- If B_{12} deficiency: vitamin B_{12}, 100 mcg IM × 5 days, then 100 mcg IM every mo

- Loperamide, 2–4 mg PO tid–qid (max: 16 mg/day), or kaolin/pectin (Kaopectate), 60–90 mL PO qid PRN

- Solu-Medrol, 10–20 mg IV q6h, *or* prednisone, 40–60 mg PO daily *or*

  Hydrocortisone, 100 mg IV q6h

- Asacol, 400–800 mg PO tid–qid, *or* 5-aminosalicylate, 400–800 PO tid/enema 4 g/60 mL PR qh *or*

  Sulfasalazine, 0.5–1g PO q6h, *or* olsalazine, 500 mg PO bid, *or* mesalamine 1 g PO q6h *or*

  Hydrocortisone retention enema: 100 mg in 120 mL saline bid

SYMPTOMS

TABLE 3–9: Diagnosis: Acute Abdominal Pain	
Disposition	Medical floor
Monitor	Vitals
Diet	NPO
Fluid	MIVF
O_2	PRN
Activity	?Bedrest
Dx studies	
Labs	CBC, BMP, Ca^+, Mg^+, LFT, bilirubin, PT/PTT/INR, amylase, lipase, β-HCG if female
	UA, lactic acid, blood C&S, urine C&S, ?troponin, ?hepatitis panel
	?Toxicology screen, ?serum acetaminophen level
Radiology and cardiac studies	CXR (PA and lateral) (pneumonia, perforation)
	US of abdomen: gallstones, ovarian cyst if female, ectopic pregnancy, hydronephrosis, ascites
	Flat-plate/acute abdominal series: renal stones, perforation, impaction
	CT (abdominal/pelvic): malignancy, pseudocyst, abscess, appendicitis, aortic dissection
	?Colonoscopy: malignancy, IBD, ischemic bowel disease

(continued)

TABLE 3–9: Diagnosis: Acute Abdominal Pain (Continued)	
Special tests	?*C. difficile* toxin A and B (if antibiotic use in past 1 mo)
	?Upper endoscopy: gastritis, PUD
	?Upper GI series with small bowel follow-through (barium vs. gastrografin)
	?ERCP: stone in bile duct
	?Manual cervical examination if female: PID, STD (GC and chlamydia Cx, wet mount/KOH)
	?Bladder scan: urinary retention (BPH, prostate cancer)
	?Laparotomy: malignancy, uterine fibroid, adhesions (history of previous surgery)
	?Celiac disease: IgA endomysial antibody or IgA tissue transglutaminase antibody
Prophylaxis	DVT
Consults	?GI, ?surgery
Nursing	Stool guaiac, NG tube if small bowel obstruction suspected, I/O
Avoid	?
Management	Treat underlying etiology
Etiologies of Abdominal Pain	

Right upper quadrant	Left upper quadrant
Cholecystitis/cholangitis	Pelvic inflammatory disease if female
Intussusceptions	Ovarian cyst if female
Pancreatitis	Diverticulosis

(continued)

TABLE 3–9: Diagnosis: Acute Abdominal Pain (Continued)

Right upper quadrant	Left upper quadrant
Hepatitis/hepatomegaly	Intussusceptions
Ischemic bowel	Ischemic bowel
Intestinal perforation	Intestinal perforation
MI	MI
Pneumonia empyema/ pleurisy	Pancreatitis
Gastritis/PUD	Pneumonia
Renal stones	Gastritis/PUD
Herpes zoster	Renal stone
Pericarditis	Herpes zoster
Retrocecal appendicitis	Splenic injury/infarct/abscess
Subdiaphragmatic abscess	Empyema
Acetaminophen overdose	
Budd-Chiari syndrome	
Right lower quadrant	**Left lower quadrant**
Appendicitis	Intussusceptions
Intussusceptions	Diverticulitis
Renal stone/nephrolithiasis	IBD (Crohn's or UC)
Intestinal perforation	Ischemic bowel
Ischemic colitis	Renal stone
Herpes zoster	Intestinal perforation
Psoas abscess	Irritable bowel syndrome
IBD (Crohn's or UC)	Herpes zoster

(continued)

TABLE 3–9: Diagnosis: Acute Abdominal Pain (Continued)

Right lower quadrant	Left lower quadrant
Irritable bowel syndrome	Psoas abscess
Mesenteric adenitis	Epididymitis (males)
Inguinal hernia	Seminal vesiculitis (males)
Seminal vesiculitis (males)	Ectopic pregnancy (females)
Epididymitis (males)	Endometriosis (females)
Endometriosis (females)	Ovarian causes (females)
Salpingitis (females)	Salpingitis (females)
Ovarian causes (females)	
Ectopic pregnancy (females)	
PID (females)	
Epigastric	**Generalized**
Gastritis/GERD/PUD	Peritonitis
Pancreatitis	Gastroenteritis
Hernia	Intestinal obstruction
MI	Fecal impaction
Pericarditis	Intestinal perforation
Ischemic bowel	Ischemic bowel disease
Intestinal perforation	Irritable bowel syndrome
Pneumonia	Porphyria
Esophageal rupture (Boerhaave's syndrome)	Metabolic/DKA/uremia
AAA rupture	Sickle cell crisis
Periumbilical	Pancreatitis
Early appendicitis	Adhesions from previous surgery

(continued)

TABLE 3–9: Diagnosis: Acute Abdominal Pain (Continued)	
Periumbilical	**Generalized**
Gastroenteritis	Trauma
Bowel obstruction	Malaria
AAA rupture	Leukemia
Mesenteric adenitis	Mesenteric adenitis
Adhesions from previous surgery	Mesenteric thrombosis
Miscellaneous causes of abdominal pain	AAA rupture
Toxins (lead poisoning)	Sepsis
Narcotic withdrawal	CHF
Herpes zoster	Sickle cell anemia
Hypersensitivity reaction	Psychogenic
Acute adrenal insufficiency	
Henoch-Schönlein purpura	

TABLE 3–10: Diagnosis: Diarrhea with or without Abdominal Pain

Disposition	Medical floor, ?monitor bed if electrolyte disturbance
Monitor	Electrolyte monitoring
Diet	NPO except ice chips (if no diarrhea for ≥12 hrs → consider placing patient on clear fluid)
Fluid	Correct deficit with NS, then D_5NS or D_5 1/2 NS for maintenance
O_2	PRN
Activity	Bedrest
Dx studies	
Labs	CBC with differential, BMP, calcium (pancreatic insufficiency), Mg, PO_4, LFT
	Stool leukocyte, ova and parasite, stool C&S, stool guaiac, UA, blood C&S
Radiology and cardiac studies	Abdominal x-ray (flat-plate and upright)
	CT of abdomen: ischemic colitis
Special tests	?*C. difficile* toxin A and B, ?HAV-IgM, β-HCG if female
	Stool for electrolytes to calculate stool osmolar gap to differentiate osmolar vs. secretory
	Stool Cx: Lab should be notified of *Aeromonas* and *Yersinia*
	Stool Cx for *Salmonella* and *Shigella*, stool Wright's stain for leukocyte
	?IgA endomysial antibody or IgA tissue transglutaminase antibody for celiac disease

(continued)

TABLE 3–10: Diagnosis: Diarrhea with or without Abdominal Pain (Continued)	
Prophylaxis	DVT
Consults	?GI (endoscopy if IBD suspected), ?surgery
Nursing	I/O, stool guaiac
Avoid	Loperamide hydrochloride (Imodium) if *C. difficile* suspected
Management	
PPI *or* H$_2$ blocker	
Note	
Consider not using any Kaopectate, Imodium, or Lomotil until etiology determined	
If *C. difficile* suspected → start treatment empirically before Cx results	
• Kaopectate: 1,200–1,500 mg PO after loose bowel movement *or*	
• Imodium: 2 capsules PO initially *or*	
• Lomotil: 2 tablets or 10 mL PO qid *or*	
• Psyllium hydrophilic mucilloid (Metamucil): 1–2 tablets with juice *or*	
• Sucralfate (Carafate), 1 g PO 1 hr before meal and qh	

TABLE 3–11: Diagnosis: GI Bleeding (Upper or Lower)	
Disposition	Medical floor/unit if hemodynamically unstable
Monitor	Vitals
	Cardiac monitoring
Diet	NPO
Fluid	Initially resuscitate NS/LR (wide open to 125 mL/hr), then place on MIVF
	IV access: 2 large-bore (14–18), blood transfusion if low H&H
O_2	≥2 L O_2 via NC; keep O_2 saturation >92%
Activity	Bedrest
Dx studies	
Labs	H&H q2–4h initially, then q4–8h CBC, BMP, Mg, PO_4
	Type and cross 2–4 PRBC and 2–4 units FFP, NG aspirate guaiac
	LFT, PT/PTT/INR, fibrinogen
Radiology and cardiac studies	EGD, portable CXR (PA and lateral), flat-plate of abdomen
	ECG, colonoscopy, ?upper GI series with small bowel follow-through
Special tests	?Radionucleotide imaging, enteroclysis*
	?Ammonia, ?Meckel scan
	?RBC scan (technetium 99m scan), ?angiography, ?capsule endoscopy
Prophylaxis	?
Consults	GI, surgery, interventional radiology

(continued)

TABLE 3–11: Diagnosis: GI Bleeding (Upper or Lower) (Continued)	
Nursing	I/O, NG tube (to evaluate upper GI bleeding in patients with hematochezia); monitor urine output
Avoid	Heparin, warfarin (Coumadin), NSAIDs, ASA, steroids

Management

- Transfuse 2–6 units PRBC if profuse bleeding or low H&H

- Pantoprazole (Protonix): 80 mg IV over 15 min, then 8 mg/hr or 40 mg IV bid *or*

  Ranitidine, 50 mg IV q6–8h, *or* famotidine, 20 mg IV q12h

- If high INR → vitamin K, 10 mg IV/SQ daily, and have FFP, 2–4 units, ready

- Variceal bleed

  Octreotide: 25–50 mcg IV bolus followed by continuous IV infusion of 25–50 mcg/hr *or*

  Vasopressin: 20 units IV over 20–30 min → 0.2–0.3 units/min for 30 min → ↑ by 0.2 units/min until bleeding stops (max: of 0.9 units/min)

  Nitroglycerin paste, 1 inch q6h off qh, or nitroglycerin, 10–30 mcg/min infusion (50 mg in 250 D_5W)

*Enteroclysis: a double-contrast study performed by passing a tube into the proximal small bowel and injecting barium and methylcellulose; it is superior to standard imaging with small bowel follow-through for identifying other lesions such as small bowel tumors, ulcers, and Crohn's disease. Enteroclysis can also be performed with CT scanning (CT enteroclysis).

4
Hematology/Oncology

TABLE 4–1: Diagnosis: DVT	
Disposition	Cardiac monitor bed
Monitor	Vitals
Diet	Regular
Fluid	Heplock (flush every shift)
O_2	PRN
Activity	Bedrest with elevation of extremity involved
Dx studies	
Labs	CBC, BMP, calcium, LFT, PT/PTT/INR, ABG, UA, urine R&M
Radiology and cardiac studies	CXR (PA and lateral), venous Doppler US, CT of chest, ?V/Q scan, ECG
	MRI from inferior vena cava to popliteal veins
Special tests	Coagulation panel (coagulation panel labs may vary from lab to lab), ?malignancy workup
	Protein C&S, antithrombin III, anticardiolipin antibody, factor V Leiden
	Plasminogen, antiphospholipid antibodies, lupus anticoagulant, ?ANA
Prophylaxis	?
Consults	?Hematology/oncology
Nursing	Measure circumference of the area involved, stool guaiac
Avoid	IM injections

(continued)

TABLE 4–1: Diagnosis: DVT (Continued)
Management
• Warm packs to area involved (for pain control)
• Heparin: bolus 80–100 units/kg IV, then 18–20 units/kg/hr; check PTT 6 hr after starting infusion (PTT 1.5–2.0 control)
or
• Enoxaparin (Lovenox): 1 mg/kg SQ q12h/1.5 mg/kg SQ daily (check factor Xa)
• Start warfarin, 5–10 mg PO daily, when PTT is therapeutic
• Overlap heparin or Lovenox and warfarin for at least 3–4 days and when INR has been between 2–3 for 2 consecutive days, then discontinue heparin
• Pain management (see Chapter 12, Table 12–21)
• Docusate (Colace): 100 mg PO qh for constipation

TABLE 4–2: DVT Prevention

Medical conditions

- Heparin: 5,000 units SQ q12h

- Enoxaparin (Lovenox): 40 mg SQ once daily; if CrCl <30 mL/min → 30 mg SQ daily

- Dalteparin (Fragmin): 2,500 units SQ once daily

- Nadroparin*: 2,850 units SQ once daily

General surgery in moderate-risk patient

- Heparin: 5,000 units SQ q12h

- Enoxaparin: 20 mg SQ 1–2 hrs before surgery and daily after surgery

- Dalteparin: 2,500 units SQ 1–2 hrs before surgery and daily after surgery

- Nadroparin*: 2,850 units SQ 2–4 hrs before surgery and daily after surgery

- Tinzaparin (Innohep): 3,500 units SQ 2 hrs before surgery and daily after surgery

General surgery in high-risk patient

- Heparin: 5,000 units SQ q8h or q12h

- Enoxaparin (Lovenox): 40 mg SQ 1–2 hrs before surgery and daily after surgery or 30 mg SQ q12h starting 8–12 hrs after surgery

- Dalteparin (Fragmin): 5,000 units SQ 8–12 hrs before surgery and daily after surgery

Orthopedic surgery

- Heparin is not recommended

- Enoxaparin: 30 mg SQ q12h starting 12–24 hrs after surgery or 40 mg SQ daily starting 10–12 hrs after surgery

- Dalteparin: 5,000 units SQ 8–12 hrs before surgery, then daily starting 12–24 hrs after surgery or 2,500 units SQ 6–8 hrs after surgery, then 5,000 units SQ daily

(continued)

TABLE 4–2: DVT Prevention (Continued)

- Nadroparin*: 38 units/kg SQ 12 hrs before surgery; 12 hrs after surgery; and once daily on postoperative days 1, 2, and 3; then ↑ to 57 units/kg SQ daily

- Tinzaparin: 75 units/kg SQ daily starting 12–24 hrs after surgery; or 4,500 units SQ 12 hrs before surgery and daily after surgery

Major trauma

- Heparin: 5,000 units SQ q8h

- Enoxaparin: 30 mg SQ every 12 hrs (for acute spinal cord injury)

- Enoxaparin: 30 mg SQ every 12 hrs starting 12–36 hrs after injury if the patient is hemodynamically stable

*Not approved.

TABLE 4–3: Diagnosis: Sickle Cell Crisis	
Disposition	Unit
Monitor	Vitals
Diet	Regular
Fluid	IVF is essential but promote PO intake as much as possible
O_2	≥ 2 L O_2 via NC; keep O_2 saturation >92%
Activity	Bedrest
Dx studies	
Labs	CBC with differential, BMP, LFT, blood C&S, UA, urine C&S, reticulocyte count, parvovirus titer
	Unsure of diagnosis: check Howell-Jolly bodies on peripheral smear and hemoglobin electrophoresis
Radiology and cardiac studies	CXR (PA and lateral), ?CT of chest
Special tests	Type and cross PRBC, LDH, bilirubin (direct and indirect), haptoglobin, direct Coombs'
Prophylaxis	DVT, pneumococcal vaccine polyvalent (Pneumovax), and influenza vaccine
Consults	Hematology/oncology
Nursing	Stool guaiac
Avoid	?
Management	
Note: If hemolysis, ↑ lactate dehydrogenase, ↑ indirect bilirubin, ↓ haptoglobin	

(continued)

TABLE 4–3: Diagnosis: Sickle Cell Crisis (Continued)
Pain management
• Ketorolac tromethamine (Toradol): 30–60 mg IV/IM q6h PRN *or*
• Acetaminophen (Tylenol #3): 1–2 tablets PO q4–6h PRN *or*
• Morphine: 5–10 mg IV/IM/SQ q2–4h PRN *or*
• Meperidine (Demerol): 50–150 mg IV/IM q4–6h PRN *or*
• Hydroxyzine pamoate (Vistaril): 25–100 mg IV/IM/PO q4h PRN
Supportive care
• Ondansetron (Zofran): 4 mg IV/PO q4–6h PRN for N/V
• Zolpidem (Ambien): 5–10 mg PO qh for insomnia
• Folic acid: 1 mg PO daily
• *Haemophilus influenzae* vaccine: 0.5 mL IM
• Pneumococcal vaccine: 0.5 mL IM
• Hydroxyurea: 15 mg/kg/day (max: 35 mg/kg/day), ↑ 5 mg/kg/day q12weeks

5
Infectious Disease*

---

*See Guide Tables: Antibiotic Spectrum for information on antibiotics.

TABLE 5–1: Diagnosis: Cellulitis	
Disposition	Medical floor
Monitor	Vitals
Diet	Regular
Fluid	Heplock (flush every shift)
O₂	PRN
Activity	PRN
Dx studies	
Labs	CBC with differential, blood C&S × 2, BMP
Radiology and cardiac studies	X-ray of the site of cellulitis, ?CT scan, ?MRI, ?technetium/gallium bone scan
Special tests	?Wound Cx, ?skin biopsy, ?sinus drainage/?aspirate Cx, ?ESR
Diagnosing cellulitis associated with hemolytic streptococci group A, C, or G	Antistreptolysin-O
	Antideoxyribonuclease B
	Antihyaluronidase
Prophylaxis	DVT
Consults	?ID, ?skin/wound care
Nursing	Warm compresses (Curity heater), keep affected area elevated if possible
Avoid	?
Management	Urgent surgery required for necrotizing fasciitis; see Management: Cellulitis
	Consider whirlpool therapy

(continued)

TABLE 5–1: Diagnosis: Cellulitis (Continued)

Management: Cellulitis

- Cefazolin: 1 g IV q6–8h first line
- Nafcillin: 1.0–1.5 g IV q4–6h first line
- Ceftriaxone: 1 g IV q24h first line
- Cefazolin, 2 g IV q24h, plus probenecid, 1 g PO daily first line

If MRSA or PCN allergy

- Vancomycin: 1–2 g IV daily first line
- Linezolid: 0.6 g IV q12h first line

Patient can be switched to oral medication once patient is afebrile and resolution of cellulitis is noted

- Dicloxacillin: 0.5 g PO q6h first line
- Cephradine: 0.5 g PO q6h first line
- Cephalexin: 0.5 g PO q6h first line
- Cefadroxil: 0.5–1.0 g PO q12–24h first line

Source: Reprinted from Morton N, Swartz, MD. Clinical practice. Cellulitis. *N Engl J Med* 2004;350:9, with permission.

(continued)

TABLE 5–1: Diagnosis: Cellulitis (Continued)
Management of Cellulitis Associated with Specific Condition
• PCN allergy: erythromycin, 500 mg PO q6h
• Human bite: amoxicillin/clavulanate (Augmentin) or cefoxitin IV
• Animal bite: PCN IV or nafcillin IV or cefoxitin IV
• Facial cellulitis: cefotaxime IV; if oral cavity involved, cover anaerobes with clindamycin/metronidazole (Flagyl)
• Diabetic patient: cefoxitin or clindamycin plus gentamicin
• IV drug abuse: vancomycin plus gentamicin
• Burn patient: vancomycin plus gentamicin
• Compromised patient: clindamycin plus gentamicin
• Suspicion of anaerobe: clindamycin, 600 mg IV q8h, or metronidazole, 500 mg IV q6h
• Gas-forming infection: clindamycin, 600 mg IV q8h, or metronidazole, 500 mg IV q6h

TABLE 5–2: Diagnosis: *Clostridium difficile (C. difficile)*	
Disposition	Medical floor/surgical floor; isolation precaution
Monitor	Vitals
Diet	Regular
Fluid	Heplock (flush every shift)
O$_2$	PRN
Activity	?Up ad lib in the room
Dx studies	
Labs	CBC with differential
Radiology and cardiac studies	?CT of abdomen
Special tests	*C. difficile* toxin A and B
Prophylaxis	?
Consults	?ID
Nursing	?
Avoid	Antidiarrhea agents
Management	
• Metronidazole: 500 mg PO tid or 250 mg PO/IV qid × 10–14 days first line	
• Vancomycin: 125 mg PO qid × 10–14 days (IV not effective) second line	
• Bacitracin: 25,000 units PO qid × 10–14 days third line	
• Cholestyramine: 4 g PO tid × 10–14 days (use in addition to above antibiotics for relapsing *C. difficile*)	
Note: Add *Saccharomyces boulardii* (Florastor), one 250-mg tablet PO bid for recurrent *C. difficile*	

TABLE 5–3: Diagnosis: Diverticulitis	
Disposition	Medical floor/surgical floor
Monitor	Vitals
Diet	NPO; advance to clear diet when tolerated
Fluid	Heplock (flush every shift)
O₂	PRN
Activity	?Bedrest
Dx studies	
Labs	CBC with differential, BMP, LFT, blood C&S × 2
Radiology and cardiac studies	Acute abdominal series, CT of abdomen
Prophylaxis	DVT
Consults	?Surgery, ?GI
Nursing	NG tube to intermittent low suction is obstructed
Avoid	?
Management	

• Consider placing patient on clear liquid/NPO

Mild (treat for 7–10 days)

• TMP/SMX DS PO bid first line

• Ciprofloxacin: 750 mg PO bid first line

• Levofloxacin (Levaquin), 750 mg PO daily, plus metronidazole, 500 mg PO q6h first line

• Amoxicillin/clavulanate ER 1,000/62.5 mg 2 tablets PO bid second line

Mild to moderate

• Piperacillin/tazobactam (Zosyn): 3.375 g IV q6h or 4.5 g IV q8h first line

(continued)

TABLE 5–3: Diagnosis: Diverticulitis (Continued)
• Ampicillin/sulbactam (Unasyn): 3 g IV q6h first line
• Ticarcillin/clavulanate (Timentin): 3.1 g IV q6h first line
• Ertapenem: 1 g IV daily first line
• Ciprofloxacin: 400 mg IV q12h second line
• Levofloxacin, 750 mg IV q24h, plus metronidazole, 500 mg IV q6h second line
Severe
• Imipenem/cilastatin (Primaxin): 500 mg IV q6h first line
• Meropenem: 1 g IV q8h first line
• Ampicillin, 2 g IV q6h, plus metronidazole, 500 mg IV q6h, plus ciprofloxacin, 400 mg IV q12h second line
• Ampicillin, 2 g IV q6h, plus metronidazole, 500 mg IV q6h, plus levofloxacin, 750 mg IV q24h second line
• Ampicillin, 2 g IV q6h, plus metronidazole, 500 mg IV q6h, plus gentamicin or amikacin second line

TABLE 5–4: Diagnosis: Endocarditis	
Disposition	?Unit/monitor floor
Monitor	Vitals
	Cardiac monitoring
	Neuromonitoring
Diet	Regular
Fluid	Heplock (flush every shift)
O_2	PRN
Activity	Up ad lib
Dx studies	
Labs	CBC with differential, BMP, calcium, Mg, LFT, blood C&S (four sets over 24 hrs), UA, urine C&S
Radiology and cardiac studies	TEE, ECG, CXR (PA and lateral)
Special tests	?Pulmonary V/Q scan useful in right-sided endocarditis
	CT of chest for locating abscess
	Serology of *Chlamydia* and *Bartonella* in Cx-negative endocarditis
	?ESR, ?C_3, C_4, CH_{50}, ?CRP
Prophylaxis	?
Consults	?Surgery, ?ID, ?cardiology
Nursing	?
Avoid	?
Management	See Management: Endocarditis

(continued)

TABLE 5–4: Diagnosis: Endocarditis (Continued)	
Duke Criteria for Infective Endocarditis (IE)	
2 Major criteria *or* 1 major plus 3 minor criteria *or* 5 minor criteria	
Major criteria	**Minor criteria**
1. Positive blood Cx	1. Fever ≥38°C (100.4°F)

A. Atypical organism associated
     with IE
	2. History of heart
	   condition or IV drug use

• *Streptococcus viridans,* *Streptococcus bovis*	3. Microbiologic evidence

• HACEK*	A. Positive blood Cx
	     but does not meet
	     major criteria

B. *S. aureus* or enterococci in the absence of primary focus	*or*

2. Persistently positive blood Cx	B. Serologic evidence
	     of active evidence
	     with organism
	     consistent with IE

A. Defined as two positive blood Cx >12 hrs apart	4. Vascular phenomenon
B. All three or a majority of four Cx (first and fourth 1 hr apart)	A. Major arterial emboli
3. Positive echocardiogram	B. Septic pulmonary infarct
A. Oscillating intracardial mass on valve or supporting structure	C. Mycotic aneurysm

B. Abscess	D. Conjunctival/
	     intracranial
	     hemorrhage

C. New partial dehiscence of prosthetic valve	E. Janeway lesion

(continued)

TABLE 5–4: Diagnosis: Endocarditis (Continued)	
Major criteria	**Minor criteria**
4. New murmur	5. Immunologic phenomenon
	A. Glomerulonephritis
	B. Osler's node
	C. Roth's spots
	D. Rheumatoid factor
	6. Echocardiographic finding that does not meet major criteria

Haemophilus species (*H. parainfluenzae*, *H. aphrophilus*, and *H. paraphrophilus*), *Actinobacillus actinomycetemcomitans*, *Cardiobacterium hominis*, *Eikenella corrodens*, and *Kingella* species

Source: Reproduced from Durack DT, Lukes AS, Bright DK. New criteria for diagnosis of infective endocarditis: utilization of specific echocardiographic findings. Duke Endocarditis Service. *Am J Med* 1994;96:200–209, with permission.

Von Reyn Criteria for Diagnosis of IE

Definite IE

1. Direct evidence by histology, bacteriology, valvular vegetation, or peripheral emboli

Probable IE

1. Persistently positive blood Cx plus one of the following:

   A. New regurgitant murmur

   B. Predisposing heart disease or vascular phenomenon

2. Negative or intermittently positive blood Cx plus the following:

   A. Fever

   B. New regurgitant murmur

   C. Vascular phenomenon (i.e., splinter/conjunctival hemorrhage, petechiae, Roth's spots, emboli)

(continued)

TABLE 5–4: Diagnosis: Endocarditis (Continued)

Possible IE

  1. Persistently positive blood Cx plus one of the following:

    A. Predisposing heart disease (exclude permanent heart disease)

    B. Vascular phenomenon

  2. Negative or intermittently positive blood Cx plus the following:

    A. Predisposing heart disease

    B. Vascular phenomenon

    C. Fever

Management: Endocarditis

- Streptococci: PCN, 2–4 million units IV q4h, plus gentamicin × 2 weeks[a]

  Note: Use only PCN × 4 weeks in patients with renal insufficiency or cranial nerve VIII damage

- Enterococci: PCN, 5–10 million units IV q4h, plus gentamicin/streptomycin × 4–6 weeks[a]

- Staphylococcus (native valve): oxacillin or nafcillin, 2 g IV q4h × 6 weeks (use gentamicin for initial 3–5 days)

- Staphylococcus (prosthetic valve): vancomycin, 15 mg/kg IV infused over 1 hr q12h × 6 weeks, plus rifampin, 300 mg PO q8h × 6 weeks, plus gentamicin for first 2 weeks

- HACEK organisms: ceftriaxone, 2 g IV/IM q24h × 4 weeks

If PCN allergy

PCN-susceptible streptococci

- Vancomycin, 15 mg/kg IV over 1 hr q12h, plus gentamicin for 4–6 hrs[b]

- Ceftriaxone, 2 g IV/IM × 4 weeks[c] *or*

- Ceftriaxone, 2 g IV, plus gentamicin, 3 mg/kg daily, × 2 weeks[a]

(continued)

TABLE 5–4: Diagnosis: Endocarditis (Continued)
Enterococci
• Consider PCN desensitization
• Vancomycin, 15 mg/kg IV over 1 hr q12h, plus gentamicin × 4–6 weeks[a,b]
Staphylococcus (native valve)
• Cefazolin, 2 g IV q8h[c]
• Vancomycin, 15 mg/kg IV over 1 hr q12h × 6 weeks[b]

[a]Patient with prosthetic valve treat for 6 weeks.
[b]Vancomycin, usual dose 1 g over 1 hr q12h.
[c]Consider not using in patient with type I hypersensitivity.

TABLE 5–5: Diagnosis: HIV Management

Disposition	Medical floor/?unit
Monitor	Vitals
	Cardiac monitoring
	Neuromonitoring
Diet	Regular
Fluid	Heplock (flush every shift)
O$_2$	PRN
Activity	Bedrest/?isolation
Dx studies	
Labs	CBC with differential, BMP, Mg, calcium, LFT
Radiology and cardiac studies	CXR (PA and lateral), ?CT of head
Special tests	Total lymphocyte count (TLC),* CD4
Prophylaxis	See Prophylactics
Consults	ID
Nursing	?
Avoid	?
Management	See treatment tables on following pages

*TLC can be used as proxy for CD4 when combined with clinical symptoms.
TLC <1,200/µL = CD4 <200 cells/µL

Prophylactics

CD4 count	Condition/organism	Regimen
<200 cells/µL	PCP	TMP/SMX
		Dapsone
		Atovaquone

(continued)

TABLE 5–5: Diagnosis: HIV Management (Continued)

CD4 count	Condition/organism	Regimen
	S. pneumoniae	Pneumococcal vaccine polyvalent (Pneumovax)
	Coccidioidomycosis	Fluconazole
<100 cells/μL	*Toxoplasma gondii*	TMP/SMX
		Dapsone
		Atovaquone
	Histoplasmosis	Itraconazole
<50 cells/μL	*Mycobacterium avium* complex	Clarithromycin
		Rifabutin
	Cryptococcosis	Fluconazole
		Itraconazole
	CMV	Ganciclovir

HIV Treatment Guidelines: International AIDS Society-USA Guidelines for Starting Antiretroviral Therapy

Symptomatic HIV	Treatment needed
Asymptomatic plus CD4 <200 cells/μL	Treatment needed
Asymptomatic plus CD4 >200 cells/μL	Treatment needed for following:
	CD4 200–350 cells/μL
	CD4 rate of decline >100 μL/yr
	Viral load >50,000–100,000 copies/mL

Source: From Yeni PG, Hammer SM, Carpenter CC, et al. Antiretroviral treatment for adult HIV infection in 2002: updated recommendations of the International AIDS Society-USA Panel. *JAMA* 2000;288:222, with permission.

(continued)

TABLE 5–5: Diagnosis: HIV Management (Continued)		
Initial Regimen: Department of Health and Human Services Guidelines		
Select one from column A and one from column B		
	A	**B**
Preferred	Efavirenz (EVF)	Stavudine (d4T)/ lamivudine (3TC)
	IDV	Zidovudine (AZT)/ didanosine (ddI)
	Nelfinavir (NFV)	AZT/3TC
	Ritonavir (RTV)/ saquinavir (SQV) (Fortovase)	d4T/ddI
	RTV/indinavir (IDV)	ddI/3TC
	Lopinavir/r (LPV/r)	
Alternative	Abacavir (ABC)	AZT/zalcitabine (ddC)
	Amprenavir (APV)	
	Delavirdine (DLV)	
	Nevirapine (NVP)	
	RTV	
	SQV	
	NFV/SQV	

(continued)

TABLE 5–5: Diagnosis: HIV Management (Continued)

Initial Regimen: International AIDS Society-USA

Preferred	Alternative
2 Nucleosides + 1 protease inhibitor ± low-dose RTV	1 protease inhibitor + nonnucleoside reverse transcriptase inhibitor ± 1–2 nucleoside reverse transcriptase inhibitors
2 Nucleosides + 1 nonnucleoside reverse transcriptase inhibitor	
3 Nucleosides	

Source: From Yeni PG, Hammer SM, Carpenter CC, et al. Antiretroviral treatment for adult HIV infection in 2002: updated recommendations of the International AIDS Society-USA Panel. *JAMA* 2000;288:222, with permission.

HIV Opportunistic Infection

Aspergillosis

Voriconazole: 6 mg/kg IV q12h × 1 day, then 4 mg/kg IV q12h first line

Amphotericin B: 0.7–1.4 mg/kg daily second line

Caspofungin: 70 mg IV daily, then 50 mg IV daily second line

Bartonella henselae and *Bartonella quintana*

Erythromycin: 500 mg PO qid first line

Doxycycline: 100 mg PO bid second line

Azithromycin: 0.5–1.0 g PO daily second line

Doxycycline, 100 mg PO bid, plus rifampin, 300 mg IV/PO bid

Candida species

Esophagitis

Fluconazole: 200 mg PO daily first line

(continued)

TABLE 5–5: Diagnosis: HIV Management (Continued)
Itraconazole: 200 mg PO daily (take on an empty stomach) second line
Voriconazole: 200 mg PO bid
Caspofungin: 70 mg IV q24h × 1 day, then 50 mg IV q24h
Thrush
Clotrimazole oral troches: 10 mg 5 × a day first line
Nystatin: 500,000 units; gargle 4–5 times a day second line
Fluconazole: 100 mg PO daily second line
Itraconazole: 100-mg oral suspension; swish and swallow daily second line
Amphotericin B: 0.3–0.5 mg/kg IV daily second line
Vaginitis
Butoconazole 2% cream: apply daily first line
Clotrimazole 1% cream: apply daily first line
Miconazole 2% cream: daily or 100-mg vaginal suppository apply daily first line
Ketoconazole: 200 mg PO bid
Coccidioides immitis (coccidioidomycosis)
Pulmonary or disseminated
Amphotericin B: 0.5–1.0 mg/kg IV q24h with or without fluconazole
Meningitis
Fluconazole: 400–800 mg PO daily first line
Itraconazole: 200–400 mg PO bid second line
Cryptococcus neoformans
Meningitis
Amphotericin B, 0.7 mg/kg IV daily, plus 5-fluorocytosine, 100 mg/kg PO daily first line

(continued)

TABLE 5–5: Diagnosis: HIV Management (Continued)

Fluconazole, 400–800 mg PO daily, plus 5-fluorocytosine, 100 mg/kg PO daily second line

Amphotericin B (AmBisome): 4 mg/kg IV daily second line

Pulmonary or disseminated

Fluconazole: 200–400 mg PO daily first line

Itraconazole: 200 mg PO bid (take on an empty stomach) second line

Cryptosporidium parvum

HAART (highly active antiretroviral therapy) first line

Nitazoxanide: 500 mg PO bid third line

Paromomycin, 1 g PO bid, plus azithromycin, 600 mg PO daily third line

Atovaquone: 750-mg suspension PO bid with meal third line

CMV

Retinitis

Ganciclovir implant q6mo plus valganciclovir, 900 mg PO bid first line

Ganciclovir: 5 mg/kg IV bid first line

Foscarnet: 60 mg/kg IV q8h or 90 mg/kg q12h first line

Valganciclovir: 900 mg PO bid

Cidofovir, 5 mg/kg IV twice a week, plus probenecid, 2 g PO q3h second line

Extraocular disease (GI: esophagitis or colitis)

Valganciclovir: 900 mg PO bid first line

Ganciclovir: 5 mg/kg IV bid first line

Foscarnet: 60 mg/kg q8h or 90 mg/kg IV q12h first line

(continued)

TABLE 5–5: Diagnosis: HIV Management (Continued)
Neurologic disease
Ganciclovir, 5 mg/kg IV bid, plus foscarnet, 90 mg/kg IV bid first line
Ganciclovir: 5 mg/kg IV bid second line
Pneumonitis
Ganciclovir: 5 mg/kg IV bid first line
Foscarnet: 60 mg/kg q8h or 90 mg/kg IV q12h first line
Valganciclovir: 900 mg PO bid first line
Entamoeba histolytica
Metronidazole, 750 mg IV/PO tid, plus diiodohydroxyquin, 650 mg PO tid, plus paromomycin, 500 mg PO tid first line
Paromomycin: 500 mg PO tid second line
Haemophilus influenzae
Cefuroxime first line
TMP/SMX second line
Second- or third-generation cephalosporin second line
Fluoroquinolones second line
Herpes simplex
Labialis
Acyclovir: 400 mg PO tid; severe: 5–10 mg/kg IV q8h first line
Famciclovir: 500 mg PO bid first line
Valacyclovir: 1 g PO bid first line
Penciclovir topical: q2h (use in conjunction with valacyclovir, famciclovir, or acyclovir) first line
Pneumonitis, esophagitis, hepatitis, or dissemination
Acyclovir: 5–10 mg/kg IV q8h
Encephalitis
Acyclovir: 10 mg/kg IV q8h

(continued)

TABLE 5–5: Diagnosis: HIV Management (Continued)

Herpes zoster

  Dermatomal

    Famciclovir: 500 mg PO tid first line

    Valacyclovir: 1 g PO tid first line

    Acyclovir: 30 mg/kg IV daily first line for severe disease

  Ophthalmic or visceral involvement

    Acyclovir: 30–36 mg/kg IV daily for first line

    Foscarnet: 40 mg/kg IV q8h or 60 mg/kg q12h second line

  Chickenpox

    Acyclovir: 10 mg/kg IV q8h or 800 mg PO qid first line

    Valacyclovir: 1 g q8h second line

Histoplasma capsulatum

    Amphotericin B: 0.7 mg/kg IV daily first line

    AmBisome: 3–5 mg/kg IV daily first line

    Fluconazole: 800 mg PO daily second line

***Isospora belli* (isosporiasis)**

    TMP/SMX: two DS PO bid or one DS tid first line

    Pyrimethamine, 50–75 mg PO daily, plus leucovorin acid, 5–10 mg PO daily

JC virus (progressive multifocal leukoencephalopathy)

    HAART first line

    Interferon alpha: 3 MU daily second line

    Cidofovir plus HAART second line

***Microsporidia* (microsporidiosis)**

    Enterocytozoon bieneusi: fumagillin (Fumidil B), 60 mg PO daily (may cause neutropenia and thrombocytopenia) first line

    Encephalitozoon intestinalis: albendazole, 400 mg PO bid first line

(continued)

TABLE 5–5: Diagnosis: HIV Management (Continued)
Ocular: Fumidil B, 3 mg/mL saline eye drops first line
Metronidazole: 500 mg PO tid second line
Nitazoxanide: 500 mg PO bid (currently in an experimental stage) third line
***M. avium* complex**
Clarithromycin, 500 mg PO bid, plus ethambutol (EMB), 15 mg/kg PO daily first line
Azithromycin, 500–600 mg PO daily, plus EMB, 15 mg/kg PO daily first line
Severe symptoms
Above two drugs plus ciprofloxacin, 500–750 mg PO bid first line
Above two drugs plus levofloxacin, 500–750 mg PO daily first line
Above two drugs plus rifabutin, 300 mg PO daily first line
Mycobacterium chelonae
Clarithromycin: 500 mg PO bid first line
Cefoxitin or amikacin or doxycycline or imipenem or erythromycin or tobramycin second line
Mycobacterium fortuitum
Amikacin, 400 mg IV q12h, plus cefoxitin, 1–2 g IV daily
Mycobacterium kansasii
Isoniazid (INH), 300 mg PO daily, plus rifampin, 600 mg PO daily, plus EMB, 25 mg/kg daily, ± streptomycin, 1 g IM
Ciprofloxacin, 750 mg PO bid, plus clarithromycin, 500 mg PO bid
Mycobacterium scrofulaceum
Surgical excision first line

(continued)

TABLE 5–5: Diagnosis: HIV Management (Continued)

Mycobacterium tuberculosis

INH plus rifampin plus pyrazinamide (PZA) plus EMB × 8 weeks, then INH plus rifampin × 18 weeks first line

INH plus rifabutin plus PZA plus EMB × 8 weeks, then INH plus rifabutin × 18 weeks second line

Latent tuberculosis

INH, 300 mg PO daily, plus pyridoxine, 50 mg PO daily first line

INH, 900 mg PO twice a week, plus pyridoxine, 50 mg PO twice a week first line

Nocardia asteroides

Trisulfapyridine: 3–12 g PO daily first line

TMP/SMX: 5–15 mg/kg PO daily first line

Minocycline: 100 mg PO bid second line

Penicillium marneffei

Amphotericin B: 0.7–1.0 mg/kg IV daily first line

Itraconazole: 200 mg PO bid

P. carinii

TMP, 15 mg/kg PO daily, plus SMX, 75 mg/kg PO/IV daily first line

Hypoxemia: Add prednisone 40 mg PO bid

TMP, 15 mg/kg PO daily, plus dapsone, 100 mg PO daily second line

Pentamidine: 3–4 mg/kg IV q24h second line

Clindamycin, 600–900 mg IV q6–8h, plus primaquine, 15–30 mg PO daily second line

Atovaquone: 750-mg suspension PO bid second line

Pseudomonas aeruginosa

Aminoglycoside plus antipseudomonal β-lactam first line

Antipseudomonal β-lactam second line

(continued)

TABLE 5–5: Diagnosis: HIV Management (Continued)
Carbapenem second line
Ciprofloxacin second line
Aminoglycoside second line
Salmonella **spp.**
Ciprofloxacin: 500 mg PO bid first line
TMP 1 DS PO bid second line
S. aureus
MSSA
Nafcillin or oxacillin ± gentamicin 1 mg/kg IV q8h first line
Cephalexin: 500 mg PO qid first line
Dicloxacillin: 500 mg PO qid first line
Clindamycin: 300 mg PO tid first line
Fluoroquinolone first line
First-generation cephalosporin ± gentamicin or rifampin second line
MRSA
Vancomycin, 1 g IV q12h, ± gentamicin or rifampin first line
Linezolid: 600 mg PO/IV bid
Streptococcus pneumoniae
PCN or amoxicillin or cefotaxime, ceftriaxone, or fluoroquinolone first line
Macrolide or vancomycin second line
T. gondii
Pyrimethamine, 200 mg PO loading dose, then 50–75 mg PO daily, plus leucovorin, 10–20 mg PO daily, plus sulfadiazine, 1.0–1.5 g PO q6h first line
Pyrimethamine plus leucovorin plus clindamycin, 600 mg IV q6h second line

(continued)

TABLE 5–5: Diagnosis: HIV Management (Continued)
TMP, 5 mg/kg PO bid, plus SMX, 25 mg/kg PO bid second line
5-Fluorouracil, 1.5 mg/kg PO daily, plus clindamycin, 1.8–2.4 g PO/IV bid second line
Treponema pallidum (syphilis)
Primary, secondary, and early latent syphilis (<1 yr)
Benzathine PCN G: 2.4 million units IM × 1 dose
Primary, secondary, and early latent syphilis (>1 yr or unknown)
Benzathine PCN G: 2.4 million units IM weekly × 3 weeks
Neurosyphilis
Aqueous PCN G: 18–24 million units IV daily × 10–14 days

Source: Reproduced from Bartlett J, Gallant J. *Medical management of HIV infection*. Baltimore: Johns Hopkins University Press, 2003, with permission.

TABLE 5–6: Diagnosis: Meningitis	
Disposition	Monitor floor/isolation precaution
Monitor	Vitals
	Neuromonitoring
Diet	NPO
Fluid	Heplock (flush every shift)
O$_2$	PRN
Activity	Bedrest
Dx studies	
Labs	CBC with differential, BMP, blood C&S, PT/PTT/INR, throat swab, UA, urine C&S
	CSF analysis (get CT of head before LP; see below for ordering CSF tests)
	PPD, VDRL test, rapid plasma reagent
Radiology and cardiac studies	CT of head with contrast, CXR (PA and lateral), ECG
Special tests	If nasal discharge → test for glucose and chloride to r/o CSF leak, ?HIV
	?PCR for meningococcus, ?CSF for PCR for meningococcus or viruses
	?Latex agglutination for meningococcus, pneumococcal, *H. influenzae* b
	Recurrent meningitis: Check CH$_{50}$ for terminal C6–C9
Prophylaxis	Chemoprophylaxis for exposure (see Meningococcal Infection: Chemoprophylaxis for Exposure)
Consults	ID

(continued)

TABLE 5–6: Diagnosis: Meningitis (Continued)	
Nursing	Respiratory isolation, I/O, check neurologic status q2–6h
Avoid	?
Management	See Empiric Therapy for Suspicion of Meningitis for empiric treatment
	Dexamethasone (0.15 mg/kg IV q6h)

Lumbar Puncture and Tube Contents

Tube number	Test for
1	Cell count
2	Gram stain, bacteria, viral and fungus C&S, AFB, India ink
3	Glucose, protein, LDH, VDRL test
4	Cell count, RBC count, WBC count
	Latex agglutination or counterimmunoelectrophoresis for meningococcus, pneumococcal, *H. influenzae* b, *Escherichia coli*, group B streptococcus, cryptococcal antigen, *Toxoplasma*
5	Hold for other tests

Signs and Symptoms: Meningitis

- Fever
- Headache
- Cough
- Stiff neck
- Photophobia
- Earache
- Rash
- Rhinorrhea

(continued)

TABLE 5–6: Diagnosis: Meningitis (Continued)		
• Otorrhea		
• Brudzinski's sign: Bending chin to chest can cause hips and knees flex		
• Kernig's sign: Straight-leg raising can cause pain		
Empiric Therapy for Suspicion of Meningitis		
• Antibiotic should be given empirically before LP if there is high suspicion of meningitis		
• LP can be done up to 2 hrs after first dose of empiric antibiotic therapy without destroying CSF Cx result		
Bacterial meningitis empiric treatment		
Preterm and low-weight neonate	Group B streptococcus, *Listeria monocytogenes*, *E. coli*, staphylococci, gram-negative	Vancomycin, 15 mg/kg IV q6h, plus ceftazidime (Fortaz), 50–100 mg/kg q8h
0–3 mos	Group B streptococcus, *L. monocytogenes*, *E. coli*	Ampicillin, 50 mg/kg IV q8h, plus ceftriaxone, 50–100 mg/kg IV q12h
3 mos–18 yrs	*S. pneumoniae*, *H. influenzae*, *Neisseria meningitidis*	Ceftriaxone, 50–100 mg/kg IV q12h, plus vancomycin, 10 mg/kg IV q6h
18–50 yrs immuno-competent	*S. pneumoniae*, *N. meningitidis*	Ceftriaxone, 2 g IV q12h, plus vancomycin, 500 mg IV q6h

(continued)

TABLE 5–6: Diagnosis: Meningitis (Continued)		
>50 yrs immuno-competent	S. pneumoniae, L. monocytogenes, gram-negative bacilli	Ampicillin, 2 g IV q4h, plus ceftriaxone, 2 g IV q2h, plus vancomycin, 500 mg IV q6h
Immunocom-promised	L. monocytogenes, gram-negative bacilli	Ampicillin, 2 g IV q4h, plus ceftazidime, 50–100 mg/kg IV q8h
Head trauma, shunt, or surgery	Staphylococci, gram-negative bacilli, S. pneumoniae	Vancomycin, 15 mg/kg IV q6h, plus ceftazidime, 50–100 mg/kg IV q8h

Source: From Quagliarello VJ, Scheld WM. Treatment of bacterial meningitis. *N Engl J Med* 1997;336:708, with permission.

Meningococcal Infection: Chemoprophylaxis for Exposure	
Age	Medication
<1 mo	Rifampin: 5 mg/kg PO q12h × 2 days
>1 mo	Rifampin: 20 mg/kg PO q12h × 2 days
≤12 yrs	Ceftriaxone: 125 mg IM × 1 dose
>12 yrs	Ceftriaxone: 250 mg IM × 1 dose
Adult	Rifampin, 600 mg/kg PO q12h × 2 days, or ciprofloxacin, 500 mg PO × 1 dose

Note
Rifampin
Not recommended for pregnant female; may ↓ efficacy of oral contraceptive pills
May cause red-orange discoloration of body fluids (e.g., urine, tears)

(continued)

TABLE 5–6: Diagnosis: Meningitis (Continued)
Ciprofloxacin
Not recommended if <18 yrs of age, pregnant female, or lactating female
Can be used in children if no other alternative available

Source: From Meningococcal disease: evaluation and management of suspected outbreaks. *MMWR Morb Mortal Wkly Rep* 1997;46(RR-6):6, with permission.

TABLE 5–7: Diagnosis: Osteomyelitis	
Disposition	Medical floor
Monitor	Vitals
Diet	Regular
Fluid	Heplock (flush every shift)
O₂	PRN
Activity	Bedrest
Dx studies	
Labs	CBC with differential, blood C&S, BMP, ESR, CRP, UA, needle biopsy of bone for C&S × 2
Radiology and cardiac studies	X-ray of the site, ?CT scan, MRI (preferred), ?technetium/gallium bone scan
Special tests	?Wound Cx, ?sinus drainage/aspirate Cx, ?needle aspiration for C&S
	If patient with diabetes, consider probe to bone test
Prophylaxis	DVT
Consults	?ID, ?orthopedics
Nursing	Elevate involved area if possible
Avoid	?
Management	
• Nafcillin/oxacillin: 2 g IV q4h first line	
• Cefazolin (Ancef): 1–2 g IV q8h first line	
• Unasyn: 1.5–3.0 g IV q6h first line	
• Zosyn: 3.375–4.5 g IV q6h second line	
• Linezolid (Zyvox): 600 mg IV/PO q12h (side effect: thrombocytopenia) second line	
• MRSA suspected or PCN allergy: vancomycin, 1 g IV q12h	

(continued)

TABLE 5–7: Diagnosis: Osteomyelitis (Continued)
• Anaerobe suspected: clindamycin, 600 mg IV q6h
• Aerobes and anaerobe suspected: clindamycin plus third-generation cephalosporin or quinolone
• Diabetic or bite wound: clindamycin plus third-generation cephalosporin or quinolone
• ?Hyperbaric oxygen (not proven by randomized controlled studies)

TABLE 5–8: Diagnosis: Pelvic Inflammatory Disease (PID)	
Disposition	Medical floor
Monitor	Vitals
Diet	Regular
Fluid	Heplock (flush every shift)
O₂	PRN
Activity	Up ad lib
Dx studies	
Labs	CBC with differential, cervical Cx for GC and chlamydia, UA, urine C&S, BMP, Mg
	Blood C&S × 2, ESR, LFT
Radiology and cardiac studies	Pelvic US to r/o abscess, wet mount (NS/KOH) of vaginal secretion
Special tests	β-HCG, ?HIV, ?VDRL, ?rapid plasma reagent
Prophylaxis	?
Consults	Ob/gyn, ?ID
Nursing	?
Avoid	?

Management: PID/Salpingitis/Tuboovarian Abscess

- Doxycycline, 200 mg IV q12h × 3 days, then 100 mg IV q12h × 11 days plus

Cefoxitin, 2 g IV q6h × 2 weeks, *or* cefotetan, 2 g IV q12h × 2 weeks, *or* ertapenem, 1 g IV q24h × 3–10 days first line

- Doxycycline, 200 mg IV q12h × 3 days, then 100 mg IV q12h × 11 days plus

Ampicillin/sulbactam: 3 g IV q6h × 2 weeks second line

(continued)

TABLE 5–8: Diagnosis: Pelvic Inflammatory Disease (PID) (Continued)

- Ciprofloxacin, 400 mg IV/500 mg PO q12h, plus metronidazole, 1 g IV q24h × 2 weeks second line

- Gatifloxacin, 400 mg IV/PO q24h, plus metronidazole, 1 g IV q24h × 2 weeks second line

- Levofloxacin, 500 mg IV/PO q24h, plus metronidazole, 1 g IV q24h × 2 weeks second line

- Moxifloxacin, 400 mg IV/PO q24h, plus metronidazole, 1 g IV q24h × 2 weeks second line

- Ofloxacin, 400 mg IV/PO q12h, plus metronidazole, 1 g IV q24h × 2 weeks second line

TABLE 5–9: Diagnosis: Pneumonia	
Disposition	Medical floor
Monitor	Vitals, pulse oximeter
Diet	Regular
Fluid	Heplock (flush every shift)
O$_2$	≥2 L O$_2$ via NC; keep O$_2$ saturation >92%
Activity	Bedrest
Dx studies	Labs
	CBC with differential, BMP, Mg, LFT, blood C&S × 2, sputum Gram stain
	Sputum C&S, UA, ?ABG, ?urine C&S
Radiology and cardiac studies	CXR (PA and lateral), ECG
Special tests	?Silver stain (for *P. carinii*)
	?AFB smear and Cx, ?PPD
	?Pneumococcal PCR
	?Influenza A and B: Rapid antigen assay can distinguish between influenza A and B
	Chlamydia psittaci, Coxiella burnetii
	?*Legionella* urinary antigen (in severely ill patient)
	?Bronchoalveolar lavage
Prophylaxis	DVT
Consults	?ID
Nursing	?Isolation if suspicion of MRSA, ?pulse oximeter, aspiration precaution
Avoid	?
Management	See Management: Pneumonia for specific therapy

(continued)

TABLE 5–9: Diagnosis: Pneumonia (Continued)	
	Acetaminophen (Tylenol): 650 mg q4–6h (max: 4 g/day) PRN for temperature >38°C and pain
	NSAIDs PRN for pleuritic pain

CURB-65: Assessing Risk of Mortality and Intensive Care Admission in Patients >65 Yrs

Clinical	Points
Confusion	1
Urea ≥20 mg/dL	1
Respiratory rate	1
BP (SBP <90 mm/Hg or DBP ≤60 mm/Hg)	1
Age ≥65 yrs	1

Risk of mortality	
Score	**% Mortality**
0	0.7
1	3.2
2	13.0
3	17.0
4	41.5
5	57.0

Site of care based on CURB-65 score

• 0–1: Home treatment

• 2: Hospital or supervised home treatment

• 3–5: Hospital

• 4–5: Consider ICU

Source: Reproduced from Lim WS, van der Eerden MM, Laing R, et al. Defining community acquired pneumonia severity on presentation to hospital: an international derivation and validation study. *Thorax* 2003;58:377–382, with permission.

(continued)

TABLE 5–9: Diagnosis: Pneumonia (Continued)

PORT Criteria (Pneumonia Assessment Scale)

- If patient age ≥50 yrs → go to risk factor table and assign patient in class II–V

- If patient age <50 → assign class I to this individual

- If patient <50 yrs and has any of the following conditions or physical examination abnormalities → go to risk factor table and assign patient in class II–V; otherwise assign class I to this individual.

Conditions	Physical examination abnormality
• Active neoplastic disease	• Altered mental status
• CHF	• Pulse ≥125/min
• Chronic renal disease	• Respiratory rate ≥30/min
• Chronic liver disease	• SBP <90 mm Hg
• Cerebrovascular disease	• Temperature <35°C or >40°C

Risk factor table	Points
Demographic factors	
• Age of men	Age (yrs)
• Age of women	Age (yrs) – 10
• Nursing home resident	10
Coexisting illnesses	
• Active neoplastic disease	30
• Congestive heart failure	10
• Chronic renal disease	10
• Chronic liver disease	20

(continued)

TABLE 5–9: Diagnosis: Pneumonia (Continued)	
Risk factor table	**Points**
• Cerebrovascular disease	10
Physical examination findings	
• Altered mental status	20
• Pulse ≥125/min	10
• Respiratory rate ≥30/min	20
• SBP <90 mm Hg	20
• Temperature <35°C or >40°C	15
Lab findings	
• Arterial pH <7.35	30
• BUN ≥30 mg/dL (11 mmol/L)	20
• Sodium <130 mmol/L	20
• Glucose ≥250 mg/dL	10
• Hematocrit <30%	10
• PaO_2 <60 mm Hg	10
Radiographic findings	
• Pleural effusion	10

Disposition of patient according to the pneumonia scale			
Class	Score	Interpretation	
II	<70	Class I and II	Treat as outpatient
III	71–90	Class III	Admit for brief observation
IV	91–130	Class IV and V	Inpatient treatment
V	>130		

Source: Reproduced from Fine, Auble, Yealy, et al. A prediction rule to identify low-risk patients with community-acquired pneumonia. *N Engl J Med* 1997; 336:243, with permission.

(continued)

TABLE 5–9: Diagnosis: Pneumonia (Continued)
Management: Pneumonia

Medical ward

• No recent antibiotic therapy

    Respiratory fluoroquinolone alone *or* advanced macrolide +
       β-lactam

• Recent antibiotic use

    Advanced macrolide + β-lactam *or* respiratory fluoroquinolone
       (regimen depends on nature of recent antibiotic use)

Unit (ICU, MICU, etc.)

• Pseudomonas is not suspected

    Respiratory fluoroquinolone alone *or* advanced macrolide +
       β-lactam

• Pseudomonas is not suspected and has β-lactam allergy

    Respiratory fluoroquinolone ± clindamycin

• Pseudomonas is suspected

    Antipseudomonal agent + ciprofloxacin

    or

    Antipseudomonal agent + aminoglycoside + respiratory
       fluoroquinolone or macrolide

• Pseudomonas is suspected and has β-lactam allergy

    Aztreonam + levofloxacin

    or

    Aztreonam + moxifloxacin

    or

    Gatifloxacin ± aminoglycoside

(continued)

TABLE 5–9: Diagnosis: Pneumonia (Continued)
Nursing home
• Receiving treatment in nursing home
Respiratory fluoroquinolone alone *or* amoxicillin + advanced macrolide
Hospitalized: follow above hospitalized patient protocol

Source: Infectious Disease Society of America. Practice guideline for the management of community acquired pneumonia in immunocompetent adults, November 7, 2003, with permission.

Organisms Associated with Specific Conditions

• Alcoholism	*S. pneumoniae, P. aeruginosa,* anaerobes, gram-negative bacilli
• Aspiration	Anaerobes
• Bats or soil enriched with bird dropping	*Histoplasma capsulatum*
• Bird exposure	*C. psittaci*
• Bronchiectasis	*P. aeruginosa, Burkholderia (Pseudomonas) cepacia, S. aureus*
• COPD/smoker	*S. pneumonia, H. influenza, Moraxella catarrhalis, Legionella* spp
• Cystic fibrosis	*P. aeruginosa, B. cepacia, S. aureus*
• Farm animals or parturient cats	*C. burnetii*
• Nursing homes	*S. pneumoniae,* gram-negative bacilli, *H. influenzae, S. aureus,* anaerobes, *Chlamydia pneumoniae*
• Poor hygiene	Anaerobes
• Travel to southwestern United States	*C. immitis*

TABLE 5–10: Diagnosis: Prostatitis	
Disposition	Medical floor
Monitor	Vitals
Diet	Regular
Fluid	Heplock (flush every shift)
O$_2$	PRN
Activity	Bedrest
Dx studies	
Labs	CBC with differential, UA, urine C&S, urine R&M
Radiology and cardiac studies	?CT or US (to r/o abscess), ?transrectal US (to r/o calculi or abscess)
Special tests	?PSA
Prophylaxis	?
Consults	?Urology
Nursing	?
Avoid	?
Management	
Pain management	
• Tylenol: 650 mg PO q6h PRN for fever	
• Stool softener	
• Sitz bath	
• May consider suprapubic catheter for severe urinary retention	
Antibiotic selection	
Prostatitis (acute)	
IV agents	
• Ampicillin, 1–3 g IV divided q6h, plus gentamicin, 2 mg/kg loading dose, then 1.7 mg/kg IV q8h first line	

(continued)

TABLE 5–10: Diagnosis: Prostatitis (Continued)
• Ciprofloxacin: 400 mg IV q12h × 2 weeks first line
• Levofloxacin: 500 mg IV daily × 2 weeks first line
• Gatifloxacin: 400 mg IV daily × 2 weeks first line
• TMP/SMX: 2.5 mg/kg IV q6h × 2 weeks first line
• Aztreonam: 2 g IV q8h × 2 weeks second line
PO agents
• Ciprofloxacin XR: 1000 mg PO daily × 2 weeks first line
• Doxycycline: 200 mg PO q12h × 3 days then 100 mg PO daily × 11 days first line
• TMP/SMX SS (single strength): PO daily × 2 weeks first line
Prostatitis (chronic)
PO agents
• Ciprofloxacin: 500 mg PO bid × 1–3 mos first line
• Levofloxacin: 500 mg PO daily × 1 mo first line
• Doxycycline: 100 mg PO daily × 1–3 mos first line
• TMP/SMX DS: PO bid × 1–3 mos second line

TABLE 5–11: Diagnosis: Pyelonephritis	
Disposition	Medical floor
Monitor	Vitals
Diet	Regular
Fluid	MIVF
O₂	PRN
Activity	Up ad lib
Dx studies	
Labs	CBC with differential, BMP, Mg, LFT, UA, urine R&M, urine Gram stain and C&S
	Blood C&S × 2
Radiology and cardiac studies	KUB, renal US, CT of abdomen
Special tests	?ESR
Prophylaxis	?
Consults	?Nephrology, ?urology, ?ID
Nursing	Urine output
Avoid	?
Management	See below
	Tylenol: 325–650 mg q4–6h (max: 4 g/day)

Empiric treatment for acute uncomplicated pyelonephritis	
Parenteral	**Oral**
• Ceftriaxone: 1 g IV q24h *or*	• Ciprofloxacin: 500 mg PO bid *or*
• Ciprofloxacin: 200–400 mg IV q12h *or*	• Ciprofloxacin XR: 1,000 mg PO daily *or*
• Levofloxacin: 250–500 mg IV q24h *or*	• Levofloxacin: 250–500 mg PO daily *or*

(continued)

TABLE 5–11: Diagnosis: Pyelonephritis (Continued)	
• Ofloxacin: 200–400 mg IV q24h *or*	• Ofloxacin: 200–300 mg PO bid *or*
• Gatifloxacin: 400 mg IV q24h	• Gatifloxacin: 400 mg PO daily *or*
	• Norfloxacin: 400 mg PO bid *or*
	• Lomefloxacin: 400 mg PO daily *or*
	• Enoxacin: 400 mg PO bid

Empiric treatment for acute complicated pyelonephritis

- Cefepime: 1 g IV q12h *or*
- Ciprofloxacin: 400 mg IV q12h *or*
- Levofloxacin: 500 mg IV q24h *or*
- Ofloxacin: 400 mg IV q12h *or*
- Gatifloxacin: 400 mg IV q24h *or*
- Gentamicin, 3–5 mg/kg IV q24h, plus ampicillin, 1–2 g IV q6h *or*
- Gentamicin, 1 mg/kg IV q8h, plus ampicillin, 1–2 g IV q6h *or*
- Ticarcillin/clavulanate: 3.2 g IV q8h *or*
- Piperacillin/tazobactam: 3.375 g q6–8h *or*
- Imipenem/cilastatin: 250–500 mg q 6–8h

Empiric treatment for acute pyelonephritis in pregnancy

- Ceftriaxone: 1 g IV q24h *or*
- Gentamicin, 1 mg/kg IV q8h, plus ampicillin, 1–2 g IV q6h *or*
- Ticarcillin/clavulanate: 3.2 g IV q8h *or*
- Aztreonam: 1 g IV q8–12h *or*
- Piperacillin/tazobactam: 3.375 g q6–8h *or*
- Imipenem/cilastatin: 250–500 mg q 6–8h

TABLE 5–12: Diagnosis: Septic Arthritis		
Disposition	Medical floor	
Monitor	Vitals	
Diet	Regular	
Fluid	Heplock (flush every shift)	
O$_2$	PRN	
Activity	Up ad lib	
Dx studies		
Labs	CBC with differential, blood C&S × 2, UA, urine C&S, urine R&M, BMP, Mg	
	Male: urethral swab for GC; female: cervical swab, rapid plasma reagent/VDRL	
Radiology and cardiac studies	CXR, x-ray of the joint, CT of joint, ?technetium and gallium scintigraphic scan, ?MRI, ?indium-labeled WBC scan	
Special tests	Joint fluid analysis	
	Color	C&S	Protein
	Gram stain	WBC count	Glucose
	Viscosity	AFB	
	Blood Cx for *Neisseria gonorrhoeae*: chocolate agar or Thayer-Martin medium	
	Tuberculosis exposure: synovial fluid Cx for AFB, staining for AFB, histologic examination of the synovial membrane	
	History of trauma, animal bite, endemic fungal infection, Lyme disease, immune suppression, or refractory to conventional therapy: ?fungal Cx, ?PCR for detection of *Borrelia burgdorferi* DNA	

(continued)

TABLE 5–12: Diagnosis: Septic Arthritis (Continued)	
	?ESR, ?rheumatoid factor, ?antiteichoic acid (elevated in *Staphylococcus* infection)
	?Cryoglobulins, ?immune complexes, ?antistreptolysin-O antigen?*Brucella*- and rickettsial-related titer
	?PCR techniques to detect gonococcal DNA in synovial fluid can ↑ the yield in Cx-negative cases and permits monitoring of the response to therapy.
Prophylaxis	PRN
Consults	?ID, ?rheumatology, ?PT/OT
Nursing	Warm compresses to joint; immobilize joint involved
Avoid	Do not use tetracycline in pregnancy or children <8 yrs
Management	See Management: Septic Arthritis
P. aeruginosa is common in following conditions:	
• Patient with burn	
• Inject illicit drugs	
• Trauma, particularly after injury in aquatic environments	
• Postoperatively	
• Cellulitis in neutropenic patient	
• Chronic decubitus ulcers	
Management: Septic Arthritis	
• Arthroscopy or open drainage	
• Gram-positive cocci:	
Community-acquired infections: cefazolin, 1–2 g IV q8h	
Hospital or nursing home–acquired infection: vancomycin (30 mg/kg daily IV in two divided doses) (max: 2 g/day)	

(continued)

TABLE 5–12: Diagnosis: Septic Arthritis (Continued)
• Gram-negative bacilli:
Third-generation cephalosporin such as ceftazidime (1–2 g IV q8h) *or*
Ceftriaxone (2 g IV q24h) *or*
Cefotaxime (2 g IV q8h) *or*
P. aeruginosa suspected (e.g., in patients who inject illicit drugs):
Ceftazidime plus aminoglycoside such as gentamicin
Gram-negative pleomorphic: clindamycin
MRSA: vancomycin, 1 g IV q12h
Gonococcal suspicion: ceftriaxone, 1 g IV/IM q24h, or spectinomycin, 2 g IM q12h
• Physical therapy
• Daily aspiration
• Open débridement and lavage if no resolution with IV antibiotic and closed drainage

TABLE 5–13: Diagnosis: Septic Shock/Sepsis	
Disposition	Unit
Monitor	Vitals, continuous pulse oximeter
Diet	NPO, ?hyperalimentation
Fluid	Volume replacement then MIVF
O_2	≥ 2 L O_2 via NC; keep O_2 saturation >92%
Activity	Bedrest
Dx studies	
Labs	CBC with differential, BMP, calcium, Mg, PO_4, LFT, blood C&S $\times$ 2, UA, urine C&S
	Amylase, lipase, troponin, PT/PTT/INR, ABG, ?fungal Cx, LP, CD4, TLC
Radiology and cardiac studies	ECG, CXR (PA and lateral); KUB, ?CT of chest, ?CT of abdomen, ?CT of head, US of abdomen
Special tests	Lactic acid, serum/urine toxicology screen, ?CSF analysis, ?sputum C&S
	?Fibrinogen degradation product, fibrinogen
	?Coombs' direct/indirect (if patient receiving blood transfusion)
	?Peritoneal fluid analysis
Prophylaxis	DVT, GI prophylaxis
Consults	?ID
Nursing	Stool guaiac, Foley catheter, I/O
Avoid	?
Management	
• Resuscitation and treat hypotension (aggressive IVF, vasopressors)	
• Treat the source of septic shock	

(continued)

TABLE 5–13: Diagnosis: Septic Shock/Sepsis (Continued)

- Antibiotic therapy if infectious etiology suspected (consider broad-spectrum antibiotics)

- Neutropenia: ceftazidime, 1–2 g q8–12h, plus vancomycin

  or

  Zosyn plus gentamicin or tobramycin

  or

  Imipenem plus gentamicin or tobramycin

- Corticosteroids (stress dose: hydrocortisone, 100 mg IV q8h)

- Correction of electrolytes, give HCO_3 if pH <7.1

TABLE 5–14: Diagnosis: TB	
Disposition	Medical floor (respiratory isolation)
Monitor	Vitals
Diet	Regular
Fluid	Heplock (flush every shift)
O_2	≥ 2 L O_2 via NC; keep O_2 saturation >92%
Activity	Up ad lib in the room, ?bedrest
Dx studies	
Labs	CBC with differential, sputum for AFB, PPD, LFT, BMP, Mg, hepatitis panel
	HIV serology, anergy testing (mumps, *Candida*, and tetanus toxoid)
	Latent TB infection: serum QuantiFeron-TB Test and QuantiFeron-TB Gold Test
Radiology and cardiac studies	CXR (PA and lateral), CT of chest
Special tests	?CD4 count, ?TLC, pleural fluid analysis
	?Bone marrow biopsy to diagnose miliary tuberculosis
	Extrapulmonary: UA, urine C&S, CSF, bone marrow, and liver biopsy for Cx
Prophylaxis	?
Consults	ID, pulmonary
Nursing	Respiratory isolation
Avoid	?
Management	See Management: TB
PPD interpretation (measure induration and not erythema)	
≥5 mm of induration	
• People with HIV infection	

(continued)

TABLE 5–14: Diagnosis: TB (Continued)
• Close contacts
• People who have had tuberculosis disease before
• People who inject illicit drugs and whose HIV status is unknown
≥10 mm of induration
• Foreign-born person
• HIV-negative persons who inject illicit drugs
• Low-income groups
• People who live in residential facilities
• People with certain medical conditions
• Children younger than 4 yrs old
• People in other groups as identified by local public health officials
≥15 mm of induration
• People with no risk factors for tuberculosis
Source: From http://www.cdc.gov.
Management: TB
Direct observation therapy
First line
INH, 15 mg/kg (max: 900 mg) PO, plus rifampin, 600 mg PO plus
EMB, 30 mg/kg PO (max: 2,500 mg), plus PZA (if ≥75 kg = 3 g; if ≤50 kg = 2 g; if 51–74 kg = 2.5 g PO) three times a week for 6 mos
Second line
INH, 300 mg PO, plus rifampin, 600 mg PO, plus EMB, 15 mg/kg PO (max: 2,500 mg), plus PZA (if ≥75 kg = 2.5 g; if ≤50 kg = 1.5 g; if 51–74 kg = 2 g PO) daily for 2 mos
Then INH, 300 mg PO, plus rifampin, 600 mg PO, daily for 4 mos

(continued)

TABLE 5–14: Diagnosis: TB (Continued)
If HIV-positive
INH, 15 mg/kg (max: 900 mg) PO, plus rifampin, 600 mg PO, plus
EMB, 15 mg/kg PO (max: 2,500 mg), plus PZA (if ≥75 kg = 3 g; if ≤50 kg = 2 g; if 51–74 kg = 2.5 g PO) daily for 2 mos
Then INH, 300 mg PO, plus rifampin, 600 mg PO, daily for 7 mos
Whenever patient is on INH, he or she should be supplemented with pyridoxine, 10–50 mg PO daily

TABLE 5–15: Diagnosis: Urinary Tract Infection (UTI)	
Disposition	Medical floor
Monitor	Vitals
Diet	Regular
Fluid	IV hydration essential
O₂	PRN
Activity	Up ad lib
Dx studies	
Labs	CBC with differential, BMP, LFT, UA, urine R&M, urine Gram stain, urine C&S
	?Blood C&S
Radiology and cardiac studies	?Renal US
Prophylaxis	?
Consults	?Urology
Nursing	?
Avoid	?
Management	See below for specific treatment
	Tylenol: 325–650 mg q4–6h (max: 4 g/day)

Uncomplicated—treat for 7–10 days

• TMP/SMX DS: 1 tablet PO bid × 3 days first line

• Nitrofurantoin: 100 mg PO q12h first line

• Fosfomycin (Monurol): one 3-g packet PO × 1 dose first line

• Augmentin: 500 mg PO q12h first line

• Ciprofloxacin, 250 bid × 3 days, or ciprofloxacin, 500 daily × 3 days second line

• Levofloxacin: 250 mg PO daily × 3 days second line

• Ofloxacin: 200 mg PO bid × 3 days second line

(continued)

TABLE 5–15: Diagnosis: Urinary Tract Infection (UTI) (Continued)
• Gentamicin: 1 mg/kg IV q8h × 3 days second line
• Ticarcillin/clavulanate: 3.2 g IV q8h × 3 days second line
Complicated UTI
• Ampicillin, 1 g IV q6h, plus gentamicin, 1 mg/kg IV q8h, × 2–3 weeks first line
• Zosyn: 3.1 g IV q4–6h × 2–3 weeks second line
• Ticarcillin/clavulanate: 3.2 g IV q8h × 2–3 weeks second line
• Ceftriaxone: 1–2 g IV daily × 2–3 weeks *or*
• TMP/SMX: 800 mg PO bid × 2–3 weeks first line
• Norfloxacin: 400 mg PO bid × 2–3 weeks first line
• Ciprofloxacin: 500 mg PO bid × 2–3 weeks first line

6

Electrolyte Disturbance
and Nephrology

ELECTROLYTE DISTURBANCE

TABLE 6–1: Diagnosis: Hyponatremia	
Disposition	?Unit/medical floor (depends on level of hyponatremia)
Monitor	Vitals
	Electrolyte monitoring: Check electrolytes q4h while patient on 3% NS
	Neuromonitoring
Diet	Regular
Fluid	See below for type of fluid to be used
O_2	PRN
Activity	Bedrest
Dx studies	
Labs	Urine studies stat, BMP (q4h with rapid correction), calcium, Mg, PO_4, LFT
	TSH, uric acid, UA, serum osmolality, U_{osm}, U_{Na}, U_{Cr}
Radiology and cardiac studies	CXR (PA and lateral), ECG, ?CT of head/chest
Special tests	?Cortisol level (adrenal insufficiency), ?ADH, ?BNP (r/o CHF), ?aldosterone
	?TG level
Prophylaxis	?
Consults	Nephrology
Nursing	I/O, daily weights

(continued)

TABLE 6–1: Diagnosis: Hyponatremia (Continued)	
Avoid	• Asymptomatic patient: when correcting hyponatremia, the rate of rise in P_{Na^+} should not exceed 0.5 mEq/L/hr (12 mEq/L/24 hrs), and do not exceed P_{Na^+} 130 mEq/L
	• Symptomatic patient: initial rate of correction could be as high as 2 mEq/L/hr × 3–4 hrs → decrease to 10–12 mEq/L/day
	• Rapid correction of hyponatremia can cause central pontine myelinosis
Management	See Investigation and Management: Hyponatremia
Etiologies: Hyponatremia	
• Diuretic therapy	
• Nephropathy/ATN/nephritic syndrome	
• Adrenal insufficiency	
• Metabolic alkalosis	
• Pseudohypoaldosteronism	
• SIADH (lung disease, antidepressants, and seizure medications)	
• Third spacing (burn, ascites, effusion)	
• Glucocorticoid deficiency	
• Hypothyroidism	
• CHF	
Hyponatremia (<135)	
Pseudohyponatremia	
• Secondary to ↑ plasma glucose and high lipid and high protein contents	

(continued)

TABLE 6–1: Diagnosis: Hyponatremia (Continued)

• **Correction of Na$^+$** (glucose, protein, and TG)
• For every 100 ↑ in glucose above 200, Na$^+$ will ↓ by 1.6
• Na$^+$ deficit (mEq/L) = [plasma protein (g/L) – 8] × 0.025
• Na$^+$ deficit (mEq/L) = plasma TG (g/L) × 0.002

Note

• When correcting hyponatremia, the rate of rise in P_{Na^+} should not exceed 0.5 mEq/L/hr and should not exceed P_{Na^+} 130 mEq/L

• A major complication is **central pontine myelinolysis** (osmotic demyelination), which occurs due to rapid correction; this can be accompanied by pituitary damage and oculomotor nerve palsy. **Signs and symptoms:** diplopia, weakness, muscle spasm, paralysis, confusion, delirium, dysphagia, dysarthria

Investigation and Management: Hyponatremia

• If **hypovolemic** (patient is dry) → get U_{Na^+} level (mEq/L)

→ If U_{Na^+} >20 mEq/L → secondary to diuresis, adrenal insufficiency

→If U_{Na^+} <20 mEq/L → diarrhea, vomiting

→**Treatment**

→Symptomatic → 3% saline

→Asymptomatic → 0.9% NS (200–250 mL/hr up to 1 L, then 125–250 mL/hr)

• If **isovolemic** → differential: hypothyroidism, cortisol deficiency, thiazide, SIADH

→U_{Na^+} <10 mEq/L → water intoxication

→U_{Na^+} >20 mEq/L → SIADH, diuretic-induced

→**Treatment** → water restriction to 500–1,000 mL/day; if severe → use 3% NS

(continued)

TABLE 6–1: Diagnosis: Hyponatremia (Continued)
• If **hypervolemic** (edema) → get U_{Na^+} level (mEq/L)
→If U_{Na^+} <20 mEq/L → heart failure, cirrhosis, nephrosis
→If U_{Na^+} >20 mEq/L → renal failure
→**Treatment**
→Water restriction to 500–1,000 mL/day
→Furosemide (Lasix): 40–80 mg IV/PO daily bid
Calculating Sodium Deficit in Hypovolemic Hyponatremia
1. **Total body water (TBW)** (L): male = $[0.6 \times wt\ (kg)]$ or female = $[0.5 \times wt\ (kg)]$
2. **Na^+ concentration deficit** (mEq/L) = 130 – current Na^+ level (mEq/L)
3. **Na^+ deficit** (mEq/L) = TBW × (Na^+ concentration deficit)
4. **Fluid to be infused:** 3% saline = 513 mEq/L of Na^+, NS = 154 mEq Na^+
5. **Volume to be infused** (mL) = (Na^+ deficit/Na^+ mEq/L in solution) × 1,000
6. **Total hours for correction of sodium deficit** = Na^+ concentration deficit/0.5 [the result of this calculation is the speed of correction of Na^+ (mEq/L/hr)]
7. **Rate of infusion** = volume to be infused/hours for the infusion
Note: Do not correct the rise in P_{Na^+} to 0.5 mEq/L/hr or 12 mEq/24 hrs; correct to 130 mEq/L
Example
1. A 60-kg female with Na^+ level of 120 mEq/L
2. **TBW** (L) = (0.5 × 60) = 30 L
3. **Na^+ concentration deficit** = 130 – 120 = 10 mEq/L
4. **Na^+ deficit** (mEq/L) = (30 L) × (10 mEq/L) = 300 mEq/L
5. **Fluid to be infused:** 3% saline = 513 mEq/L of Na^+
6. **Volume to be infused** (mL) = (300/513) × 1,000 = 585 mL

(continued)

TABLE 6–1: Diagnosis: Hyponatremia (Continued)
Note: Do not correct the rise in P_{Na^+} to 0.5 mEq/L/hr or up to 130 mEq/L
7. **Total hours for correction of sodium deficit** = [(10 mEq/L)/(0.5 mEq/L)] = 20 hrs
8. **Rate of infusion** = 585 mL/20 hrs = 29 mL/hr
9. Check electrolytes q4h while patient on 3% NS

TABLE 6–2: Diagnosis: Hypernatremia	
Disposition	?Unit/medical floor (depends on level of hypernatremia)
Monitor	Vitals
	Electrolyte monitoring
	Neuromonitoring
Diet	Regular; continue oral fluids
Fluid	See below for type of fluid to be used
O_2	PRN
Activity	Bedrest
Dx studies	
Labs	BMP, calcium, Mg, PO_4, LFT, UA, serum osmolality
	Urine specific gravity, U_{osm}, U_{Na^+} and U_{K^+}, TSH
Radiology and cardiac studies	CXR (PA and lateral), ECG
Prophylaxis	?
Consults	Nephrology
Nursing	I/O, daily weights
Avoid	When correcting hypernatremia, the rate of decline in P_{Na^+} should not exceed 1 mEq/L/hr (can cause cerebral edema/herniation)
Management	See following page
Etiologies: Hypernatremia	
• Dehydration	
• Diarrhea	
• Obstructive uropathy	
• Excess sodium bicarbonate	

(continued)

TABLE 6–2: Diagnosis: Hypernatremia (Continued)
• Renal dysplasia
• Diabetes mellitus
• Diabetes insipidus (DI)
Hypernatremia (>145) (See TBW Deficit)
Hypovolemic hypernatremia
• Correct TBW deficit in 48–72 hrs
• Secondary to fluid loss → treatment: replace deficit with D_5W (see management below)
• Can give 5% albumin to rapidly restore intravascular volume
Isovolemic hypernatremia
• If secondary to DI → U_{osm} <200; if secondary to central DI → give vasopressin challenge, 5 mg IV, *or*
Desmopressin: 4 mcg IV/SQ q12h (should ↑ U_{osm} by 50%; keep urine specific gravity >1.010)
• If U_{osm} = 200–500 → nephrogenic DI → correct deficit with D_5W
• Treatment: replace TBW in 48–72 hrs
Hypervolemic hypernatremia
• Secondary to hypertonic saline solution/HCO_3 infusion/excessive salt ingestion
• Treatment: furosemide, 40–80 mg IV/PO daily–bid
• SPA (25%) 50–100 mL bid–tid
Correction of Hypovolemic Hypernatremia
1. TBW in hypernatremia: male = $0.5 \times$ wt (kg); female = $0.4 \times$ wt (kg)
2. **Current TBW** = TBW $\times [140/P_{Na^+}]$
3. **TBW deficit** = TBW − current TBW
4. **X** = replacement fluid Na^+ (mEq)/154
5. **Replacement volume** (L) = TBW deficit $\times [1/(1 - X)]$

(continued)

TABLE 6–2: Diagnosis: Hypernatremia (Continued)
Example
1. A 70-kg male with P_{Na^+} of 160 mEq/L
2. TBW = $(0.5 \times 70\ kg)$ = 35 L
3. Current TBW = $[35 \times (140/160)]$ = 30.6 L
4. TBW deficit = $(35 - 30.6)$ = 4.4 L
5. X = 75 (mEq/L)/154 = 0.49
6. Replacement volume (L) = 4.4 (L) $\times$ $[1/(1 - 0.49)]$ = 8.6 L (replace this deficit in 48–72 hrs)
Note
• Replacement: Give one-half in first 24 hrs and next half in next 48 hrs
• Isotonic fluid (NS) should be used initially if symptomatic (shock, hypotension); corrected slowly over 48–72 hrs
• The serum sodium should fall by no more than 0.5 mEq/L/hr (12 mEq/day)
• Na^+ concentration in IV fluids: NS = 154 mEq/L; $^1/_2$ NS = 75 mEq/L

TABLE 6–3: Diagnosis: Hypokalemia	
Disposition	Monitor bed
Monitor	Vitals
	Cardiac monitoring
	Electrolyte monitoring
Diet	Regular
Fluid	Heplock (flush every shift)
O$_2$	PRN
Activity	Bedrest
Dx studies	
Labs	BMP, Mg, PO$_4$, calcium, CBC, UA, LFT
Radiology and cardiac studies	ECG
Special tests	U$_{K^+}$, U$_{Cr}$, urine electrolytes, U$_{osm}$, serum osmolality
	?Renin; ?aldosterone; ?24-hr urine: K$^+$, Na, and Cr; cortisol
Prophylaxis	?
Consults	Nephrology
Nursing	I/O
Avoid	?
Management	See below

Transtubular Potassium Gradient (TTKG): Normal 8–9 (Can Be up to 12 in K$^+$-Rich Diet)

- **TTKG** = $(U_{K^+} \times P_{osm})/(P_{K^+} \times U_{osm})$

- In patient with hypokalemia without any disease, TTKG should be <3

- In patient with hypokalemia without any disease and TTKG >3, renal loss of K$^+$

(continued)

TABLE 6–3: Diagnosis: Hypokalemia (Continued)
• In patient with hyperkalemia without any disease, TTKG should be >10
• Patient with hyperkalemia and TTKG of <7 indicates hypoaldosteronism/renal tubular defect
Note
• Hypoaldosteronism: administration of mineralocorticoid 9α-fludrocortisone, 0.05 mg, should cause TTKG to rise >7
• If U_{K^+} >15 mEq/L or >30 mEq/24 hrs or TTKG >7 → renal loss
• If U_{K^+} <15 mEq/L or <25 mEq/24 hrs or TTKG <3 → extrarenal loss
Common Etiologies of Hypokalemia
• Diarrhea-/vomiting-/laxative-induced
• Pyloric obstruction
• Alkalosis
• High renin state
• True hyperaldosteronism
• Chewing tobacco
• Carbenicillin
• Mineralocorticoid [fludrocortisone (Florinef)]
• Mg depletion
• Renal tubular acidosis (RTA) I and II
• Cushing's syndrome/disease
• Adrenal hyperplasia (11β- and 17α-hydroxylase deficiency)
• Licorice
• Amphotericin B
• Diuretic (thiazide, furosemide, ethacrynic acid)
• Bartter's syndrome and Gitelman syndrome

(continued)

TABLE 6–3: Diagnosis: Hypokalemia (Continued)
Hypokalemia (<3.5 mEq)
• Check Mg level (if low, correct Mg level before correcting K^+ level)
• Mg depletion impairs K^+ reabsorption across the renal tubule
• K-Dur: 20 mEq tablet PO bid–tid
• Micro K: 10 mEq tablet PO bid–tid (max: 100 mEq/day)
• KCl elixir: 1–3 tablespoons (20 mEq in 1 tablespoon)
• 10 mEq KCl in 100 mL can be given via peripheral line over 1 hr
• 20 mEq KCl in 100 mL should be given via central line over 2 hrs
Note
• 40–60 mEq can ↑ K^+ by 1–1.5 mEq/L but this ↑ may be transient
• Do not give >10 mEq IV per hour via peripheral line or >20 mEq IV per hour via central line

TABLE 6–4: Diagnosis: Hyperkalemia	
Disposition	Monitor bed
Monitor	Vitals
	Cardiac monitoring
	Electrolyte monitoring
Diet	Low-K^+ diet
Fluid	Heplock (flush every shift)
O_2	PRN
Activity	Bedrest
Dx studies	
Labs	BMP, calcium, Mg, PO_4, LFT, CBC, serum osmolality
Radiology and cardiac studies	ECG
Special tests	U_{K^+}, U_{Na}, urine electrolytes, U_{Cr}, U_{osm}
	?Cortisol level, ?Cortrosyn stimulation test
Prophylaxis	?
Consults	Nephrology
Nursing	I/O
Avoid	See below and following pages
Management	See following pages
Common Etiologies: Hyperkalemia	
• Metabolic or respiratory acidosis	
• Adrenal insufficiency	
• Heparin	
• Insulin deficiency	
• β-Blockers	
• Arginine	

(continued)

TABLE 6–4: Diagnosis: Hyperkalemia (Continued)
• Succinylcholine
• Digitalis toxicity
• Hemolyzed blood
• Renal failure
• Aldosterone antagonist
• Hypoaldosteronism
• Blood transfusion
• Thrombocytosis/leukocytosis
• Muscle necrosis
• TMP/SMX, K^+-sparing diuretics, ACE inhibitors
TTKG: Normal 8–9 (Can Be Up to 12 in K^+-Rich Diet)
• **TTKG** = $(U_{K^+} \times P_{osm})/(P_{K^+} \times U_{osm})$
• In patient with hypokalemia without any disease, TTKG should be <3
• In patient with hypokalemia without any disease and TTKG >3, renal loss of K^+
• In patient with hyperkalemia without any disease, TTKG should be >10
• Patient with hyperkalemia and TTKG of <7 indicates hypoaldosteronism/renal tubular defect
Note
• Hypoaldosteronism: administration of mineralocorticoid 9α-fludrocortisone, 0.05 mg, should cause TTKG to rise >7
Causes of Hyperkalemia That Do Not Respond to Mineralocorticoid Challenge
• K^+-sparing diuretics
Amiloride

(continued)

TABLE 6–4: Diagnosis: Hyperkalemia (Continued)
Spironolactone
Triamterene
• Drugs
Trimethoprim
Pentamidine
• Tubular resistance to aldosterone
Interstitial nephritis
Sickle cell disease
Urinary tract obstruction
Pseudohypoaldosteronism type I
• ↑ Distal nephron K^+ reabsorption
Hyperkalemia (Recheck K^+ Level and Get ECG) → If K^+ >7, ECG Changes, or Symptomatic → Consider Treatment
• Secondary to
Transcellular shift: acidosis/myonecrosis
Blood transfusion (1 unit of whole blood can ↑ K^+ by 0.25 mEq/ 24 hrs)
Medications: ACE inhibitors, heparin, NSAIDs, digitalis, β-blockers, TMP/SMX, K^+-sparing diuretics
• Check U_{K^+} level
If >30 mEq/L → suggests transcellular shift
If <30 mEq/L → suggests impaired renal secretion
• **Treatment**
• Calcium gluconate: 10 mL of 10% (1 ampule); infuse slowly over 2–3 mins (onset 2–3 mins)
• Repeat dose in 5 min if ECG changes persist

(continued)

TABLE 6–4: Diagnosis: Hyperkalemia (Continued)
• Insulin (regular): 10 U + 50 mL of a 50% glucose solution IV (onset 15–20 mins)
• Bicarbonate: 45 mEq (1 amp of 7.5% $NaHCO_3$) IV over 5 mins (onset 30 mins); effective only in setting of metabolic acidosis
• Albuterol: 10–20 mg in 4 mL saline by nasal inhalation over 10 mins (onset 30 mins)
• Na^+ polystyrene (Kayexalate): 20–30 g with 100 mL of 20% sorbitol PO q4–6h
• To give Kayexalate as enema: 50 g in 50 mL of 70% sorbitol plus 150 mL tap water
• If no response to above treatment or severe hyperkalemia → consider dialysis

TABLE 6–5: Diagnosis: Hypomagnesemia	
Disposition	Medical floor
Monitor	Vitals
	Cardiac monitoring
	Electrolyte monitoring
	Neuromonitoring
Diet	Regular
Fluid	Heplock (flush every shift)
O_2	PRN
Activity	Bedrest
Dx studies	
Labs	BMP, Mg, calcium, PO_4, CBC
Radiology and cardiac studies	ECG
Special tests	24-hr urine Mg, urine Mg, urine electrolytes, U_{Cr}
Prophylaxis	?
Consults	?Nephrology
Nursing	?
Avoid	?
Management	See Management: Hypomagnesemia (<1.8 mg/dL)

(continued)

TABLE 6–5: Diagnosis: Hypomagnesemia (Continued)		
Etiologies: Hypomagnesemia (<1.8 mg/dL)		
Urinary loss	**Intestinal loss**	**Miscellaneous**
• Hypercalcemia	• Malabsorption	• Alcoholism
• Hyperglycemia	• Laxative use	• Sepsis
• Hypophosphatemia	• Pancreatitis	• Malnutrition
• RTA	• Severe diarrhea	• Metabolic acidosis
• Bartter's syndrome and Gitelman syndrome	• Intestinal and biliary fistula	• Hungry bone syndrome
• Novel paracellin-1 mutation		• Thermal injury
Medications		• Hyperthyroidism
• Aminoglycosides	• Digitalis	• Diabetes
• Amphotericin B	• Diuretics	• Hypoalbuminemia
• β-Agonist	• Foscarnet	• TPN
• Cisplatin	• Insulin	• Citrated blood product
• Catecholamine	• Pentamidine	
• Cyclosporine		
Management: Hypomagnesemia (<1.8 mg/dL)		
• Mg deficit = 0.2 × wt (kg) × desired ↑ in Mg concentration → replace within 2–3 days		
• **Note:** Monitor respiratory drive and tendon reflexes when replacing Mg		
• **Treatment**		
• MgOx: 400 or 600 mg PO (600 mg provides 35 mEq) 1–2 tablets daily		

(continued)

TABLE 6–5: Diagnosis: Hypomagnesemia (Continued)
• MgCl: 65–130 mg PO tid–qid (64 mg = 5.3 mEq/tablet)
• Severe (<1 mg/dL): MgSO$_4$, 1–6 g in 500 mL D$_5$W at 1 g/hr
Note: Sulfate can cause metabolic acidosis if used for a long period of time

TABLE 6–6: Diagnosis: Hypermagnesemia	
Disposition	Medical floor
Monitor	Vitals
	Cardiac monitoring
	Electrolyte monitoring
	Neuromonitoring
Diet	Regular
Fluid	Heplock (flush every shift)
O_2	PRN
Activity	Bedrest
Dx studies	
Labs	BMP, Mg, calcium, PO_4, CBC
Radiology and cardiac studies	ECG
Special tests	24-hr urine Mg, urine Mg, urine electrolytes, U_{Cr}
Prophylaxis	?
Consults	?
Nursing	?
Avoid	?
Management	See below
Hypermagnesemia (>2.3)	
• Check ECG ($\uparrow$ PR, $\uparrow$ QRS)	
• **Treatment**	
• Saline diuresis → NS or $^1/_2$ NS at 100–300 mL/hr	
• Calcium chloride (CaCl): 1–3 g in IVF at 1 g/hr	
• Furosemide: 20–40 mg IV q4–6	
• If Mg >9 → stat hemodialysis	

TABLE 6–7: Diagnosis: Hypocalcemia	
Disposition	?Monitor bed/medical floor
Monitor	Vitals
	Cardiac monitoring
	Electrolyte monitoring
	Neuromonitoring
Diet	Regular (salt deficient)
Fluid	Heplock (flush every shift)
O$_2$	PRN
Activity	Bedrest
Dx studies	
Labs	CBC, BMP, calcium, Mg, PO$_4$, intact PTH, LFT
Radiology and cardiac studies	ECG, CXR (PA and lateral)
Special tests	?24-hr urine calcium, Mg, PO$_4$, and K$^+$
Prophylaxis	?
Consults	?
Nursing	?
Avoid	Caffeine
Management	See below
Calcium (8.8–10.3 mg/dL; 4.4–5.2 mEq/L; 2.2–2.6 mmol/L)	
• ↓ Albumin 1 g = ↓ calcium 0.8 mg/dL (0.2 mmol/L)	
• Corrected [calcium] = measured total [calcium] mg/dL + [0.8 × (4 − [albumin] g/dL)]	
Etiologies: Hypocalcemia	
• Hypoalbuminemia	• Hyperphosphatemia

(continued)

TABLE 6–7: Diagnosis: Hypocalcemia (Continued)		
• Hypomagnesemia	• Recent use of MRI with gadolinium, which can lead to pseudohypocalcemia	
• Excess fluoride	• Vitamin D deficiency	
• Hypoparathyroidism	• Pancreatitis	
• **Drugs**		
Ethylenediaminetetraacetic acid (EDTA)		Bisphosphonate
Cisplatin		Foscarnet
Leucovorin		Cinacalcet
Citrate		
• Large volume of blood transfusion (citrate used as an anticoagulant chelates calcium)		
Symptoms: Hypocalcemia		
• Paresthesia		
• Hypotension		
• Chvostek's sign		
• Bradycardia		
• Prolongation of QT interval		
• Tetany		
• Seizure		
• Trousseau's sign		
• Cardiac contractility		
Management: Hypocalcemia		
Acute treatment		
• CaCl 10% (270 mg calcium/10 mL vial): give 5–10 mL over 10 mins		
• CaCl 10% (270 mg calcium/10 mL vial): dilute in 50–100 mL D_5W over 20–30 mins		

(continued)

TABLE 6–7: Diagnosis: Hypocalcemia (Continued)
• Calcium gluconate: 20 mL of 10% (2 vials): infuse over 10–15 mins followed by infusion of 60 mL in 500 mL of D_5W at 0.5–2 mg/kg/hr
Chronic treatment
• Calcium carbonate (Oscal), 1–2 tablets PO tid; calcium citrate (Citracal), 1 tablet PO q8h
• Vitamin D_2 (ergocalciferol), 1 tablet PO daily; calcitriol, 0.25 mcg PO daily, titrate up to 0.5–2 mcg qid (in chronic kidney disease)
• Docusate sodium (Colace): 1 tablet PO bid

TABLE 6–8: Diagnosis: Hypercalcemia	
Disposition	?Monitor bed/medical floor
Monitor	Vitals
	Cardiac monitoring
	Electrolyte monitoring
	Neuromonitoring
Diet	Regular (calcium restriction 400 mg/24 hrs)
Fluid	IVF hydration essential before starting diuresis
O_2	PRN
Activity	Up ad lib
Dx studies	Labs
Labs	CBC, BMP, LFT, Mg, PO_4, TSH, total ionized calcium
Radiology and cardiac studies	CXR, ECG, female: ?mammogram
Special tests	Intact PTH, 25-OH vitamin D, PTH-related protein, 24-hr calcium and PO_4, male: ?PSA
Prophylaxis	?
Consults	?Endocrine
Nursing	Seizure precaution, I/O, neuro check q2–6h
Avoid	?
Management	See Management: Hypercalcemia
Etiologies: Hypercalcemia	
↑ **Bone resorption**	
• Hyperparathyroidism (primary and secondary)	
• Malignancy	
• Hyperthyroidism	

(continued)

TABLE 6–8: Diagnosis: Hypercalcemia (Continued)
• Paget's disease
• Tamoxifen
• Hypervitaminosis A
↑ **Calcium absorption**
• Milk alkali syndrome
• Hypervitaminosis D (lymphoma, sarcoidosis)
Miscellaneous
• Lithium
• Thiazide diuretics
• Rhabdomyolysis
• Theophylline toxicity
• Adrenal insufficiency
• Familial hypocalciuric hypercalcemia
• Metaphyseal chondroplasia (very rare)
• Congenital lactase deficiency (very rare)
Management: Hypercalcemia
• IVF: NS at 200–300 mL/hr, then adjust to maintain the urinary output to 100–150 mL/hr, followed by furosemide, 10–20 mg IV
• Zoledronic acid (Zometa): 4 mg IV over 15 mins
• Pamidronate (Aredia): 60–90 mg IV over 4 hrs q24h (if Ca^+ >13.5 mg/dL)
• Etidronate: 7.5 mg/kg/24h IV daily × 3 days or (alendronate: 5–10 mg PO qd or 70 mg PO weekly)
• Calcitonin: 4–8 IU/kg IM/SQ q6h if NS and Lasix not effective
• Hydrocortisone: 200 mg IV daily × 3 days
• Plicamycin (Mithracin): 25 mcg per kg per day IV over 6 hrs for 3–8 doses
• Gallium nitrate (Ganite): 100–200 mg per m^2 IV over 24 hrs for 5 days
• Dialysis

TABLE 6–9: Diagnosis: Hypophosphatemia	
Disposition	Medical floor
Monitor	Vitals
	Electrolyte monitoring
Diet	Regular
Fluid	Heplock (flush every shift)
O_2	PRN
Activity	Up ad lib
Dx studies	
Labs	CBC, BMP, Mg, PO_4, calcium, LFT, PTH, albumin
Radiology and cardiac studies	ECG, CXR
Prophylaxis	?
Consults	?Nephrology
Nursing	?
Avoid	?
Management	See Management: Hypophosphatemia (<2.3 mg/dL)
Etiologies: Hypophosphatemia	
• Acute respiratory alkalosis	
• Phosphate binders	
• Hyperparathyroidism	
• Primary renal phosphate wasting	
• Malnutrition	
• Fanconi's syndrome	
• Vitamin D deficiency	
• Hyperglycemia	

(continued)

TABLE 6–9: Diagnosis: Hypophosphatemia (Continued)
Management: Hypophosphatemia (<2.3 mg/dL)
• If >1
→ Neutra-Phos capsule: 2 250-mg tablets PO bid or tid
→ Phospho-Soda: 5 mL PO bid or tid (5 mL = 129 mg phosphorus)
• If <1
→ Na phosphate or K^+ phosphate: 0.08–0.16 mmol/kg over 6 hrs until phosphorus level is 1.5 mg/dL
→ Na phosphate or K^+ phosphate: 10 mmol in 250 mL NS or D_5W over 8 hrs
Note: Rapid replacement with phosphorus can cause hypocalcemia (monitor for signs: tetany)

TABLE 6–10: Diagnosis: Hyperphosphatemia	
Disposition	Medical floor
Monitor	Vitals
	Electrolyte monitoring
Diet	Regular (phosphorus-deficient)
Fluid	Heplock (flush every shift)
O₂	PRN
Activity	Up ad lib
Dx studies	
Labs	BMP, Mg, PO₄, calcium, LFT, PTH, albumin
Radiology and cardiac studies	CXR (PA and lateral), ECG
Prophylaxis	?
Consults	?Nephrology
Nursing	?
Avoid	Calcium citrate, aluminum-containing products
Management	See Management: Hyperphosphatemia (>4.3 mg/dL)
Etiologies: Hyperphosphatemia	
• Ketoacidosis	
• Lactic acidosis	
• Tumor lysis syndrome	
• Rhabdomyolysis	
• Acromegaly	
• Hypoparathyroidism	
• Phosphate supplements (Fleet enema/bowel preparation laxatives with Na phosphate)	

(continued)

TABLE 6–10: Diagnosis: Hyperphosphatemia (Continued)
Management: Hyperphosphatemia (>4.3 mg/dL)
Mild to moderate
• Calcium carbonate: 1 g with each meal
• Calcium acetate (PhosLo): 1–3 667-mg tablets with each meal
• Insulin and glucose (cell phosphate uptake) used when rapid ↓ in phosphate needed
• Aluminum hydroxide (Amphojel): 5–10 mL or 1–2 tablets PO ac tid
• Aluminum carbonate (Basaljel): 5–10 mL or 1–2 tablets PO ac tid
Severe
• NS: 1–3 L over 1–3 hrs
• Acetazolamide (Diamox): 500 mg PO or IV q6h
• Dialysis

TABLE 6–11: Diagnosis: Metabolic Acidosis (Gap or Non-Anion Gap)	
Disposition	Monitor bed/?unit
Monitor	Vitals
	Cardiac monitoring
	Electrolyte monitoring
	Neuromonitoring
Diet	NPO
Fluid	Heplock (flush every shift)
O_2	≥2 L O_2 via NC; keep O_2 saturation >92%
Activity	Bedrest
Dx studies	
Labs	CBC with differential, BMP, Mg, calcium, PO_4, LFT, plasma acetone, ETOH level
	Blood C&S, UA, ?urine C&S, serum/urine toxicology screen, plasma osmolality
Radiology and cardiac studies	CXR (PA and lateral)
Special tests	?Methanol level, ?paraldehyde level, ?salicylate level, ?ethylene glycol level, lactic acid level (see Etiologies: Increased Lactic Acid Level), osmolal gap
Prophylaxis	?
Consults	?
Nursing	I/O, stool guaiac
Management	Treat underlying cause
Avoid	?

(continued)

TABLE 6–11: Diagnosis: Metabolic Acidosis (Gap or Non-Anion Gap) (Continued)
Note
Think of MUD PILES:
• **M**ethanol
• **U**remia
• **D**iabetic ketoacidosis
• **P**araldehyde
• **I**ron, isoniazid
• **L**actic acid
• **E**thanol, ethylene glycol
• **S**alicylates
Anion gap may be normal in methanol or ethylene glycol intoxication if there is concurrent ETOH ingestion
Anion gap (10–14 mEq/L) = $Na^+ - (Cl^- + HCO_3^-)$
Anion gap decreases 2.5 mEq per 1 g/dL albumin drop
Etiologies: Increased Anion Gap Metabolic Acidosis
• Lactic acidosis
• Ketoacidosis
• Methanol
• Ethylene glycol
• Rhabdomyolysis
• ASA
• Toluene
• Paraldehyde/phenformin
• Renal failure (uremia)
• Iron/isoniazid

(continued)

TABLE 6–11: Diagnosis: Metabolic Acidosis (Gap or Non-Anion Gap) (Continued)

Etiologies: Increased Lactic Acid Level

- Regional hypoperfusion

- Severe hypoxemia

- Diabetes

- Liver disease

- Sepsis

- Pheochromocytoma

- Shock (cardiogenic, septic, or hypovolemic)

- Severe anemia

- Carbon monoxide poisoning

- Malignancies

- Thiamine deficiency

Osmolal Gap

- Osmolal gap = measured osmolality – calculated osmolality

- Calculated osmolality = $[2 \times (Na^+) + (glucose/18) + (BUN/2.8) + (ethanol/4.6)]$

- Increased osmolal gap in methanol and ethylene glycol

- Also increased in ethanol, sorbitol, isopropyl alcohol, and mannitol but patient not acidotic

NEPHROLOGY

TABLE 6–12: Diagnosis: Acute Renal Failure	
Disposition	Medical floor
Monitor	Vitals
	Cardiac monitoring
	Electrolyte monitoring
	Neuromonitoring
Diet	Renal diet (not necessary if patient already on dialysis)
Fluid	Fluid challenge if prerenal azotemia suspected
	IVF should not contain K^+, Mg^+, or phosphate
O_2	PRN
Activity	Bedrest
Dx studies	
Labs	CBC with differential, BMP, calcium, Mg, PO_4, UA, urine R&M, CrCl
	Urine C&S, LFT, uric acid; CPK level if rhabdomyolysis suspected
Radiology and cardiac studies	Renal US, CXR, ECG
Special tests	?Urine electrolytes, U_{Cr}, U_{osm}, urine eosinophils
	?ESR, ?CRP, blood C&S
	?Inflammatory disorders: ANA, anti-DS DNA, ANCA, anti-GBM antibodies, complement level

(continued)

TABLE 6–12: Diagnosis: Acute Renal Failure (Continued)	
	Cryoglobulin, rheumatoid factor (cryoglobulin screen), hepatitis C antibody
	?Serum and urine electrophoresis, ?24-hr urine protein, Cr, and Na^+
Prophylaxis	?
Consults	Nephrology, ?urology (if postrenal failure suspected)
Nursing	Foley catheter, I/O, stool guaiac, ?daily weight
Avoid	ACE inhibitors, ARBs, NSAIDs, contrast dye, Mg-containing products
	Drugs associated with interstitial nephritis (see Drugs Associated with Interstitial Nephritis)
Management	Treat etiology

Note: Bacitracin can cause pseudo Cr elevation

Etiologies: Acute Renal Failure	
Prerenal	**Postrenal**
• Dehydration	• BPH
• Shock	• Prostate disease
• Low cardiac output	• Kidney stone
• Cirrhosis	• Pelvic malignancy
• Renal vascular disease ± ACE inhibitor/angiotensin-receptor blocker	

Intrarenal
• Prolonged renal ischemia (acute tubular necrosis)
• Medications: NSAIDs, amphotericin B, aminoglycosides

(continued)

TABLE 6–12: Diagnosis: Acute Renal Failure (Continued)

- Medications associated with interstitial nephritis (see Drugs Associated with Interstitial Nephritis)

- Contrast—AIN

- Rhabdomyolysis

- Hypercoagulable state

- Emboli

- Glomerulonephritis

Drugs Associated with Interstitial Nephritis

• Allopurinol	• NSAIDs
• Captopril	• PCN
• Cephalothin	• Phenytoin
• Cimetidine	• Pantoprazole (Protonix)
• Ciprofloxacin	• Rifampin
• Furosemide/thiazides	• TMP/SMX

Physical Examination Findings in Renal Failure

Prerenal	Intrarenal	Postrenal
Weight loss or gain	Weight gain	Enlarged prostate
Poor skin turgor	Mental status change	Weight gain
Orthostatic hypotension	Hypotension/hypertension	Bladder distention
Ascites	Increased JVD	Pelvic mass from bladder distention
Edema		

Note: Signs and symptoms include malaise, anorexia, nausea (from uremia)

(continued)

TABLE 6–12: Diagnosis: Acute Renal Failure (Continued)			
Urine Electrolytes		**Prerenal**	**Intrarenal**
U_{Na^+} (mEq/L)		<20	>30
FeNa		<1	>2
U/P_{Cr}		>40	<20
U_{osm}		>500	<35
BUN/Cr ratio		>10:1	10:1
FeNa $= (U_{Na^+}/P_{Na^+})/(U_{Cr}/P_{Cr}) \times 100$			
RTA			
Type	**I (Distal)**	**II (Proximal)**	**Hyperkalemic**
Problem	Defect in H^+ secretion	Defect in HCO_3 absorption	
Urine pH	Usually >6; never <5.3	Usually >6; can be <5.3	Usually <6
P_{K^+}	Low	Low	High
Urine NH$_4$	Low	Normal	Low
Treatment	HCO_3	$NaHCO_3/K^+$ citrate/thiazide	Diuretic/low-K^+ diet
Plasma osmolarity $(280–290) = 2 \times (Na^+) + (Glu/18) + (BUN/2.8)$			
Osmolal gap (<10) = measured plasma osmolarity by lab – calculated plasma osmolarity			

(continued)

TABLE 6–12: Diagnosis: Acute Renal Failure (Continued)	
Urine Electrolytes	
U_{Na^+} (0–300 mEq/L)	**Urine chloride (0–300 mEq /L)**
• Needed in calculating FeNa	• Useful in metabolic alkalosis
• Used in evaluation of oliguria	• Used in evaluation of volume status
High in acute tubular necrosis (usually >40)	U_{K^+} (5–300 mEq /L)
Dehydration/↓ volume status (usually <20)	• Used to determine if kidney is the source of potassium loss
• Used in evaluation of hyponatremia	• Needed to calculate TTKG
Urine osmolarity (50–1,400 Osmol/kg H_2O)	U_{Cr} (10–400 mg/dL or 0.4–2.5 g/day)
• Used in evaluation of hyponatremia	• Useful in calculating CrCl
• Used in evaluation of hyperkalemia	• Needed in calculating FeNa
• Used in evaluation of volume status	
• Needed to calculate TTKG	
Urine anion gap = [(Na$^+$) + (K$^+$)] – Cl$^-$	
• Indicated in hyperchloremic metabolic gap acidosis; negative in gastrointestinal HCO_3 loss and positive in RTA	
Note: Urine electrolytes: Normal values vary widely because they are based on individual intake of water and solute	

TABLE 6–13: Diagnosis: Nephrolithiasis	
Disposition	Medical floor
Monitor	Vitals
	Electrolyte monitoring
Diet	Regular, ?low oxalate
Fluid	Hydration is essential
O$_2$	PRN
Activity	Up ad lib
Dx studies	
Labs	CBC, BMP, calcium Mg, PO$_4$, uric acid, LFT
	UA, urine R&M, urine C&S, urine pH
Radiology and cardiac studies	KUB; IVP; ?CT of abdomen; CT urogram; US of abdomen (useful in pregnancy)
Special tests	Recover stone for chemical analysis
	PTH if elevated calcium level
	?24-hr urine: uric acid, calcium, Cr, citrate, oxalate, cystine, Na$^+$, PO$_4$, Mg$^+$
Prophylaxis	?
Consults	?Urology
Nursing	Strain urine, I/O
Avoid	Triamterene, indinavir, acetazolamide
	For oxalate stones: avoid rhubarb, peanut, spinach, tea, chocolate, cola, berries
	For cystine stones: avoid methionine-containing diet

(continued)

TABLE 6–13: Diagnosis: Nephrolithiasis (Continued)
Management
Pain management
• Hydromorphone (Dilaudid): 2–4 mg PO q4–6h PRN *or*
• Meperidine (Demerol): 75–100 mg PO q2–4h PRN *or*
• Morphine: 1–2 mg (max: 15 mg) IM/SQ or slow IV q4h PRN *or*
• Hydrocodone plus acetaminophen (5/500) (Vicodin): 1–2 tablets PO q4–6h PRN *or*
• Oxycodone plus acetaminophen (2.5/325) (Percocet): 1–2 tablets PO q6h PRN
Calcium stones
• Hydrochlorothiazide: 25–50 mg PO bid (supplement with K^+ to avoid hypokalemia) *or*
• Chlorthalidone: 25–50 mg PO qd (supplement with K^+ to avoid hypokalemia) *or*
• Indapamide: 2.5 mg PO daily *or*
• Neutral phosphate: 500 mg PO tid–qid
Uric acid stones
• Potassium citrate: 20 mEq bid (maintain urine pH = 6–7)
• Allopurinol: 300 mg PO daily
Cystine stones
• Potassium citrate to keep pH >7.5
• Tiopronin: 200–500 mg PO bid
• Penicillamine: 1–2 g PO daily
Struvite stones
• Remove stone
• Antibiotic
• Acetohydroxamic acid: 250 mg PO tid–qid

TABLE 6–14: Diagnosis: Rhabdomyolysis		
Disposition	Medical floor	
Monitor	Vitals	
	Cardiac monitoring	
	Electrolyte monitoring mainly K^+	
Diet	Regular	
Fluid	Diuresis is essential to prevent renal failure	
O_2	PRN	
Activity	Bedrest	
Dx studies		
Labs	CPK (usually >10,000 IU/L), troponin, UA, urine R&M, CBC with differential, TSH	
	BMP, calcium, Mg, PO_4 (can have ↑ potassium and phosphorus, ↓ calcium, bicarbonate, and uric acid are common with rhabdomyolysis)	
Radiology and cardiac studies	ECG	
Prophylaxis	?	
Consults	?Nephrology	
Nursing	I/O	
Avoid	IVP dye, metformin	
Management	See Management: Rhabdomyolysis	
Etiologies: Rhabdomyolysis		
• Trauma or muscle compression	• ETOH	• Extreme exertion
• Heat loss	• Sickle cell trait	• Metabolic myopathies

(continued)

TABLE 6–14: Diagnosis: Rhabdomyolysis (Continued)		
• Malignant hyperthermia	• Endocrinopathies	• Seizure
• Dermatomyositis	• Polymyositis	
Medications causing rhabdomyolysis		
• ETOH	• Cocaine	• Opioid
• Carbon monoxide	• Colchicine	• Statins
Infections causing rhabdomyolysis		
• Bacterial pyomyositis	• Influenza A and B	• Coxsackievirus
• EBV	• HSV	• Parainfluenza
• Adenovirus	• Echovirus	• HIV
• CMV	• Falciparum malaria	
Management: Rhabdomyolysis		
• Treat underlying cause		
• Fluid resuscitation with NS		
• Forced mannitol-alkaline diuresis		
• Keep pH >6		
• If compartment syndrome is suspected, compartment pressures should be measured and fasciotomy should be considered		
• Dialysis		

7
Neurology

TABLE 7–1: Diagnosis: Coma/Brain Death	
Disposition	Unit
Monitor	Vitals
	Cardiac monitoring
	Electrolyte monitoring
	Neuromonitoring/intracranial pressure monitoring if available
Diet	NPO, hyperalimentation, NG feeding
Fluid	MIVF
O₂	Ventilator support
Dx studies	
Labs	CBC with differential, BMP, LFT, Mg, PO₄, calcium, UA, ABG, serum/urine toxicology screen
	Serum acetaminophen and salicylate level, blood C&S, urine C&S
Radiology and cardiac studies	CXR (PA and lateral); ECG; CT of head, chest, abdomen, and pelvis; ?MRI of head, ?PET
Special tests	LP, CSF analysis (see below), amylase, lipase, EEG
	CSF and serum: ?neuron-specific enolase, glial protein S-100, creatine kinase, and lactate
Prophylaxis	DVT prophylaxis after ruling out intracerebral hemorrhage, GI prophylaxis if on ventilator
Consults	Ethics committee, neurology
Nursing	I/O, stool guaiac, aspiration precaution
Avoid	?

(continued)

TABLE 7–1: Diagnosis: Coma/Brain Death (Continued)		
Management		
• Manage airway		
• Assess circulation and treat with IVF or blood transfusion		
• Give thiamine before giving patient glucose		
• Treat underlying cause		
Medical Record Documentation		
1. Etiology		
2. Irreversibility of condition		
3. Absence of brainstem reflexes		
4. Absence of motor response to pain		
5. Absence of respiration with PCO_2 at least 60		
6. Justification for confirmatory test and result		
7. Result of repeat examination in 6 hrs (optional)		
Glasgow Coma Scale		
Eye opening	**Verbal response**	**Motor response**
1 = No response	1 = No response	1 = No response to pain
2 = Opens with pain	2 = Unintelligible sounds	2 = Extension with pain (decerebrate)
3 = Opens with verbal stimuli	3 = Inappropriate responses	3 = Flexion with pain (decorticate)
4 = Opens spontaneously	4 = Converse but confused	4 = Withdraws from pain stimuli
	5 = Alert and oriented	5 = Localization of pain (pushes away)
		6 = Responds to verbal commands

(continued)

TABLE 7–1: Diagnosis: Coma/Brain Death (Continued)
Brainstem reflexes (to determine brainstem function)
• Corneal reflex
• Pupillary reflex
• Gag reflex
• Doll's eye reflex
• Cold caloric test (oculovestibular reflex)
Brain Dead Criteria
Special considerations
1. Cause known
2. Cause irreversible
3. No severe overlying medical condition: electrolytes, acid–base disturbances, endocrine abnormalities
4. No drug intoxication or poisoning
5. Core temperature at least 33°C (91°F)
Clinical features
1. Unresponsiveness (no motor response to pain)
2. No grimacing to pain
3. No brainstem reflexes
a. No pupil response to light
b. No corneal reflex
c. No oculocephalic reflex (doll's eye)
d. No caloric vestibular reflex (50 mL water; allow 1 min each ear; allow 5 mins between ears)
e. No gag or cough with suction
f. No ventilatory effort
Apnea test
1. Temperature at least 36.5°C (97°F)

(continued)

TABLE 7–1: Diagnosis: Coma/Brain Death (Continued)

2. SBP at least 90

3. No diabetes insipidus or positive fluid balance in past 6 hrs

4. Preoxygenate to get PO_2 at least 200 and PCO_2 to 40 or lower

5. Shut off vent for 8 mins; stop test if respiration seen or systolic BP <90 or PO_2 significant desaturation or cardiac arrhythmia.

6. Draw ABG: Test is positive if no respiratory effort and PCO_2 is at least 60 mm Hg or there is a 20 mm Hg ↑ over baseline.

Optional confirmatory tests

1. EEG

   a. Minimum of eight scalp electrodes (interelectrode distance: 10 cm; interelectrode resistance of 100–10,000 ohms)

   b. Gains ↑ to 2 V/min

   c. Test integrity of recording system by deliberate creation of electrode artifact by manipulation

   d. Test for reactivity to pain, loud noises, or light

   e. Recording by a qualified technician for 30 mins

2. Transcranial Doppler US: absence of diastolic or reverberating flow

3. Technetium 99 HMPAO brain scan: no intracerebral uptake

4. Somatosensory evoked potentials: no response of N20–P22

5. Repeat examination in 6 hrs

LP and Tube Contents

Tube number	Test for
1	Cell count
2	Gram stain, bacteria, viral and fungus C&S, AFB, India ink
3	Glucose, protein, LDH, VDRL test
4	Cell count, RBCs, WBCs
5	Hold for other tests

TABLE 7–2: Diagnosis: Guillain-Barré Syndrome (Acute Idiopathic Demyelinating Polyneuropathy)	
Disposition	Unit
Monitor	Vitals
	Neuro check q1–4h
	Respiratory
Diet	NPO except medication if gag reflex intact
Fluid	Heplock (flush every shift)
O_2	≥2 L O_2 via NC; keep O_2 saturation >92% (monitor for respiratory depression)
Activity	Bedrest
Dx studies	
Labs	CBC with differential, BMP
Radiology and cardiac studies	CXR (AP/lateral)
Special tests	CSF analysis
Prophylaxis	DVT
Consults	Neurology, PT/OT
Nursing	Aspiration precaution
Avoid	Corticosteroids (may delay recovery)
Management	See Treatment
Etiology: Guillain-Barré Syndrome	
• Acute/subacute polyneuropathy that follows minor infective illnesses ("cold," URI), inoculations, or surgical procedures; may also occur without obvious precipitants	
• Preceding *Campylobacter jejuni* infection has been demonstrated in some cases	

(continued)

TABLE 7–2: Diagnosis: Guillain-Barré Syndrome (Acute Idiopathic Demyelinating Polyneuropathy) (Continued)

Clinical features and diagnosis

- Progressive weakness of more than one limb, with symmetric deficits; usually begins in the legs, often more proximal than distal
- Distal areflexia
- Mild sensory involvement
- Autonomic dysfunction (tachycardia, labile BP, abnormal sweating, sphincter disturbances, paralytic ileus)
- Cranial neuropathies (VII palsy)
- No fever
- Increased CSF protein (after 1 week)
- CSF white blood cell count ≤10
- Nerve conduction study: slowing of conduction (demyelination)
- Progression for up to 4 weeks
- Recovery within 4 weeks after progression stops

Treatment

Plasmapheresis:

- Three to five cycles

Intravenous immunoglobulin:

- 400 mg/kg/day for 5 days

Treatment otherwise symptomatic:

- Prevent respiratory failure or cardiovascular collapse: Patients severely affected need to be in ICU (may need elective intubation and mechanical ventilation)

Avoid corticosteroids [may delay recovery (contraindicated)]

PT/OT after acute phase

Prognosis

- 70–75% recover completely

(continued)

TABLE 7-2: Diagnosis: Guillain-Barré Syndrome (Acute Idiopathic Demyelinating Polyneuropathy) (Continued)

- 25%: mild neurologic deficits

- 5% die (respiratory failure)

- Prognosis is worse when there is evidence of previous *C. jejuni* infection, advanced age, and need for ventilatory support

TABLE 7–3: Diagnosis: Myasthenic Crisis	
Disposition	Unit
Monitor	Vitals
	Neuro check q1–4h
Diet	NPO except medication if gag reflex intact
Fluid	Heplock (flush every shift)
O$_2$	≥2 L O$_2$ via NC; keep O$_2$ saturation >92% (monitor for respiratory depression)
Activity	Bedrest
Dx studies	
Labs	CBC with differential, BMP, ABG
Radiology and cardiac studies	CXR (AP/lateral)
Special tests	Edrophonium (Tensilon) test, electromyography
	Acetylcholine receptor antibodies
Prophylaxis	?
Consults	Neurology
Nursing	Aspiration precaution
Avoid	?
Management	See Management: Myasthenic Crisis
Signs and Symptoms: Myasthenic Crisis	

Clinical syndrome: work-related weakness

• Initially, ocular muscles: Ptosis and diplopia (approximately 40%). Ultimately 90% of patients have ocular involvement.

• Then, facial and oropharyngeal muscles: dysarthria, dysphagia and facial diplegia. Occasionally, swallowing is impaired before the ocular signs appear. Virtually all patients with myasthenia gravis have some involvement of oropharyngeal and ocular muscles at some time.

(continued)

TABLE 7–3: Diagnosis: Myasthenic Crisis (Continued)

- Last, diffuse muscle weakness, worse after exertion

Electromyography

- Impaired neuromuscular transmission (decremental response with repetitive nerve stimulation or increased "jitter" and blocking of impulses with single-fiber electromyography)

Edrophonium (Tensilon) test

- Weakness improves 15–30 mins after infusion in patients with ocular signs (ptosis and strabismus), but results are more difficult to assess in patients with limb weakness or respiratory failure alone

Acetylcholine receptor antibodies

- Present in high titer in 90% of long-standing myasthenia gravis, but in only 50% of patients with ocular signs alone

Exacerbation with generalized weakness that includes respiratory muscles to the point of ventilatory failure (myasthenic crisis)

Clinically

- Restlessness, insomnia, anxiety, tachycardia, diaphoresis, and tachypnea. Later, headache, central cyanosis, hypotension, confusion and asterixis.

ABG

- PO_2 <60 mm Hg or PCO_2 >50 mm Hg demonstrates respiratory failure

Vital capacity

- If vital capacity <15 mL/kg → elective intubation is necessary to provide positive pressure ventilation

Mechanical ventilation

- Pressure support is preferred. Consider tracheostomy if intubation is needed for >2 weeks.

(continued)

TABLE 7–3: Diagnosis: Myasthenic Crisis (Continued)

Management: Myasthenic Crisis

Pharmacologic treatment

- Cholinergic drugs: Pyridostigmine (Mestinon), max dose of 120 mg every 3 hrs (by NG tube). When weaning from ventilator, restart cholinergic medications at one-half of previous dosage.

Plasma exchange

- Three to five cycles (1.5–2.0 L per exchange) until pulmonary function reaches 80% of predicted normal value (short-term benefit only)

Immunoglobulin infusion

- 400 mg/kg per day for 4–5 days. Mechanism of action is not well known (binding of receptor antibodies by the infused immunoglobulin or blockade of phagocytes that destroy the receptors?). Anecdotal evidence of clinical improvement.

- High-dose steroids: Prednisone, 60–100 mg daily, may cause transient weakness. Watch carefully.

TABLE 7–4: Diagnosis: Seizure	
Disposition	Medical floor/unit if status epilepticus
Monitor	Vitals
	Cardiac monitoring
	Electrolyte monitoring
	Neuromonitoring q1–4h
Diet	NPO
Fluid	MIVF
O_2	≥2 L O_2 via NC; keep O_2 saturation >92%
Activity	Bedrest
Dx studies	
Labs	BMP, Mg, calcium, PO_4, LFT, CBC with differential, UA
	Serum/urine toxicology screen, ETOH level
	Prolactin if patient presents within 1–2 hrs of having seizure
	If fever: blood C&S, urine C&S, sputum C&S
Radiology and cardiac studies	CXR (PA and lateral), CT/MRI of head, ECG
Special tests	ABG, LP for CSF analysis (if suspected infection or subarachnoid hemorrhage), ?RPR/?VDRL
	EEG (awake, sleep-deprived, photic stimulation, hyperventilation)
	Antiseizure medication level if patient already on medication for seizure

(continued)

TABLE 7–4: Diagnosis: Seizure (Continued)	
Prophylaxis	?
Consults	?Neurology
Nursing	Aspiration precaution, seizure precaution, low bed with rails
Avoid	Levofloxacin (Levaquin), bupropion (Wellbutrin), levothyroxine (Synthroid), amphetamine
Management	

1. Check blood glucose (fingerstick glucose); if low (<55) → thiamine, 10 mg IV, plus 1 amp of $D_{50}W$ (1 amp can ↑ glucose level by 100)

2. Management

• Bite block

• Diazepam: 5 mg/min IV [0.2 mg/kg (max: 20 mg)] *or*

Lorazepam (Ativan): 2 mg/min IV (0.1 mg/kg)

• Fosphenytoin: 1,000–1,500 (15–20 mg/kg) IV in saline or dextrose solution at 150 mg/min *or*

Phenytoin (Dilantin): 15–20 mg/kg in 100 mL NS; give loading dose of 25–50 mg/min (max: 1.5 g)

(**Note:** Do not mix phenytoin with dextrose solution; if hypotension, reduce infusion rate)

• If seizure persists → start phenobarbital, 120–260 mg IV (10–20 mg/kg)

• If seizure continues → induce coma (propofol, 1–2 mg/kg IV bolus, then 2–4 mg/kg infusion)

or

Phenobarbital: 10–15 mg/kg IV over 1–2 hrs, then 0.5–4 mg/kg/hr infusion

or

(continued)

TABLE 7–4: Diagnosis: Seizure (Continued)
Midazolam: 0.2 mg/kg IV slowly followed by 0.75–10 mcg/kg/min infusion
Patient needs intubation and ventilatory support; may need vasopressor for hypotension
3. Treat underlying cause
4. Speak to patient about revoking his or her driver's license and informing department of motor vehicles if the license has not already been revoked
Note
• Fosphenytoin loading dose for seizure: 15–20 mg/kg
• Phenytoin loading dose for seizure: 15–20 mg/kg
• **Correct Dilantin for low albumin** = (albumin × 0.2) + 0.1

TABLE 7–5: Diagnosis: Stroke (Brain Attack)	
Disposition	Unit
Monitor	Vitals
	Cardiac monitoring
	Neuro check q1–2h
Diet	NPO except medication if gag reflex intact (start diet after swallowing studies)
Fluid	MIVF (preferably without glucose)
O_2	≥2 L O_2 via NC; keep O_2 saturation >92%
Activity	Bedrest
Dx studies	
Labs	Blood glucose, CBC with differential, BMP, Mg, PO_4, LFT, PT/PTT/INR, UA
	?Serum/urine toxicology screen, fasting lipid profile
Radiology and cardiac studies	Initially, stat noncontrast CT of head, CXR
	MRI with diffuse-weighted images; very sensitive for ischemic stroke, but not required if patient is candidate for r-TPA (may delay treatment)
	?Swallowing studies, carotid duplex US, cardiac echo, ?Holter
Special tests	Lipid profile, ?ESR, ?VDRL, ?RPR, ?ANA, ?anticardiolipin antibodies
	?Lupus anticoagulant
	?Hemoglobin electrophoresis, ?coagulation panel, protein C&S

(continued)

TABLE 7–5: Diagnosis: Stroke (Brain Attack) (Continued)	
	If patient on enoxaparin (Lovenox) → ?check anti-factor Xa 4–6 hrs after first dose
Prophylaxis	DVT after ruling out intracerebral hemorrhage
Consults	Neurology, PT/OT, rehabilitation medicine, speech
Nursing	I/O, Foley catheter, above-the-knee elastic stocking, stool guaiac, aspiration precaution
	Elevate head of bed at 30–45 degrees, egg crate mattress
Avoid	?
Management	See Management: Ischemic Stroke

National Institutes of Health Stroke Scale

Description	Score	Description	Score
Level of consciousness		**Motor upper extremity [arms outstretched at 90 degrees (sitting) or 45 degrees (supine) × 10 secs]**	
Alert and responsive	0	No drift	0
Arousable to minor stimuli	1	Drift but does not fall to bed	1
Arousable to only pain stimuli	2	Some antigravity but cannot sustain	2
Unarousable/reflex responses	3	No antigravity but some movement	3
		No movement	4

(continued)

TABLE 7–5: Diagnosis: Stroke (Brain Attack) (Continued)			
Orientation		**Motor lower extremity [legs outstretched at 90 degrees (sitting) or 45 degrees (supine) × 10 secs]**	
Patient's name and current month	0	No drift	0
Patient's name or current month	1	Drift but does not fall to bed	1
Unable to state name or month	2	Some antigravity but cannot sustain	2
Commands		No antigravity but some movement	3
Open and close eyes and grip and release grip	0	No movement	4
Either of the two commands	1	**Limb ataxia, finger to nose, and heel to shin**	
Neither of the two commands	2	No ataxia	0
Gaze (horizontal extraocular muscle by voluntary or doll's eye)		Ataxia in arms or legs	1
Normal	0	Ataxia in arms and legs	2
Partial palsy	1	**Sensory (test with sharp object)**	
Forced eye deviation or total paresis	2	Normal	0
Visual field		Unilateral loss but aware of touch	1
Normal	0	Total unilateral loss	2
Quadrantanopia	1	Bilateral loss	3

(continued)

TABLE 7–5: Diagnosis: Stroke (Brain Attack) (Continued)				
Hemianopia	2	**Language**		
Blindness	3	Normal		0
Facial palsy (if stuporous check grimace)		Moderate aphasia		1
Normal	0	Severe aphasia		2
Flat nasolabial fold, asymmetric smile	1	Mute		3
Lower face paralysis (partial)	2	**Dysarthria (read set of words)**		
Complete paralysis	3	Normal		0
Neglect (touch patient on both hands simultaneously; show fingers in both visual fields)		Mild to moderate slurring		1
No neglect	0	Unintelligible or mute		2
Partial neglect (neglect in any modality)	1			
Total neglect (more than 1 modality)	2			

National Institutes of Health Stroke Scale Score and Percent with Favorable Outcome

Score		Score	
Age <60 yrs	% with favorable outcome	Age 69–75 yrs	% with favorable outcome
0–9	42%	0–9	54%
10–14	18%	10–14	27%
15–20	27%	15–20	0%
>20	12%	>20	0%

(continued)

TABLE 7–5: Diagnosis: Stroke (Brain Attack) (Continued)			
Age 61–68 yrs	% with favorable outcome	Age >75 yrs	% with favorable outcome
0–9	37%	0–9	36%
10–14	25%	10–14	15%
15–20	25%	15–20	6%
>20	0%	>20	0%

Source: From NINDS t-PA stroke study group, National Institutes of Health.

Management: Ischemic Stroke

1. Start ASA, 325 mg PO daily, ± clopidogrel (Plavix), 75 mg PO daily, if CT/MRI is negative for bleed (hemorrhagic stroke)

   • ASA plus dipyridamole (Aggrenox), 1 tablet PO bid, has been shown to be more effective than ASA for prevention of CVA

   • Alternative drug that can be used is ticlopidine, 250 mg bid, but the side effects are neutropenia, thrombocytopenia

2. Recombinant tissue plasminogen activator (rt-PA) can be used in nonhemorrhagic stroke and should present within 3 hrs, recommended by National Institute of Neurological Disorders and Stroke (see exclusion criteria below)

   • rt-PA: 0.9 mg/kg (max: 90 mg) 10% IV bolus, then give 90% over 1-hr infusion

   • Do not give ASA, heparin, or warfarin during first 24 hrs if rt-PA is given

3. Heparin and warfarin use in atherosclerotic stroke is controversial

4. Heparin and warfarin are indicated in patients with cardiogenic emboli and atrial fibrillation (keep INR = 2–3, 2.5–3.5 in mechanical valve) (see exclusion criteria below for starting patient on heparin and warfarin)

(continued)

TABLE 7–5: Diagnosis: Stroke (Brain Attack) (Continued)
5. BP management: Lowering BP in acute cerebral infarction is contraindicated unless patient has the following:
• BP: systolic >230 or diastolic >120
• Hypertensive encephalopathy is present
• Vital organs are compromised
• Cerebral ischemia secondary to aortic dissection
6. Treatment: labetalol, 10 mg IV over 1–2 mins, then repeat every 10 mins as needed, to a total dose of 150 mg (discontinue if hypotension, bradycardia, or bronchial spasm). Alternative: nicardipine IV at 5 mg/hr, ↑ by 2.5 mg/hr q5–15min to max 15 mg/hr (discontinue if hypotension, bradycardia)
7. Docusate sodium, 100 mg PO qh, *or* bisacodyl, 10–15 mg PO qh
8. Acetaminophen (Tylenol): 650 mg PO/PR q4–6h PRN for headache or temperature >38°C
9. Consider statin for cholesterol management and ACE for BP management
10. Consider ACE inhibitor, thiazide diuretic, or both for BP management and secondary stroke prevention
Note: Patient on Lovenox: may consider checking anti-factor Xa 4–6 hrs after the first dose
rt-PA Inclusion Criteria in Patient with Stroke
1. Age >18 yrs (no studies in children)
2. Clinical evidence of ischemic stroke with neurologic deficit
3. Time of onset <3 hrs; *remember*, "TIME is BRAIN"; the sooner the t-PA is given, the better the prognosis
rt-PA Exclusion Criteria in Patient with Stroke
Historical relevance
1. Stroke or head trauma within past 3 mos
2. Prior history of intracranial hemorrhage

(continued)

TABLE 7–5: Diagnosis: Stroke (Brain Attack) (Continued)
3. Any major surgery within past 14 days
4. GI or GU bleeding within past 21 days
5. MI in past 3 mos
6. Arterial puncture at noncompressible site within past 7 days
7. LP within past 7 days
Clinical relevance
8. Rapidly improving symptoms of stroke
9. Isolated or minor neurologic signs
10. Seizure at onset of stroke with postictal residual impairments
11. Symptoms suggestive of subarachnoid hemorrhage (with negative head CT)
12. Presentation consistent with acute MI or post–MI pericarditis
13. Persistent BP: systolic >185, diastolic >110
14. Pregnancy/lactation
15. Active bleeding
Relevance of lab
16. Platelets <100,000/mm^3
17. Glucose <50 mg/dL (2.8 mmol/L) or >400 mg/dL (22.3 mmol/L)
18. INR >1.7 if on warfarin
19. Elevated PTT if on heparin
Relevance of radiologic studies
20. Head CT shows evidence of hemorrhage
21. Head CT shows early infarct signs (diffuse swelling, parenchymal hypodensity, and/or effacement of >33% of middle cerebral artery territory)
Source: Report of quality standard subcommittee of American Academy of Neurology, with permission.

(continued)

TABLE 7–5: Diagnosis: Stroke (Brain Attack) (Continued)

Heparin and Warfarin Exclusion Criteria in Patient with Stroke

1. CT/MRI scan shows hemorrhage, tumor, abscess, epidural or subdural hematoma

2. Current bleeding

3. History of GI bleeding, bleeding tendencies

4. Large infarction noted on CT/MRI scan

5. Neurologic deterioration secondary to severe cerebral edema

6. Recent surgery past 14 days

7. Severe uncontrolled HTN (BP >185/110)

MRI Contraindications

Absolute contraindications	Relative contraindications
Electronically, magnetically, and mechanically activated implants:	Electronically, magnetically, and mechanically activated implants: other pacemakers, e.g.,
• Cardiac pacemakers	• For the carotid sinus
• Cardiac defibrillators	• Insulin pumps and nerve stimulators
• Ferromagnetic or electronically operated stapedial implants	• Lead wires or similar wires
• Aneurysm clips	• Carotid artery vascular clamp
• Metallic splinters in orbit	• Hemostatic CNS clips
	• Nonferromagnetic stapedial implants
	• Cochlear implants
	• Implanted bone growth/fusion stimulator

(continued)

TABLE 7–5: Diagnosis: Stroke (Brain Attack) (Continued)	
	• Prosthetic heart valves (in high fields, if dehiscence is suspected)
	• Hemostatic clips (body)
	• CHF
	• Pregnancy (claustrophobia)

TABLE 7–6: Diagnosis: Subarachnoid Hemorrhage	
Disposition	Unit
Monitor	Vitals
	Neuro check q1–4h
Diet	NPO except medication if gag reflex intact
Fluid	Heplock (flush every shift)
O$_2$	≥2 L O$_2$ via NC; keep O$_2$ saturation >92%
Activity	Bedrest
Dx studies	
Labs	BMP, Mg, calcium, CBC with differential, LFT, PT/PTT/INR, UA
Radiology and cardiac studies	Noncontrast CT of head, CXR, MRI (see contraindications below), ECG
	MRI/MRA: sensitive for acute ischemic lesions, presence of vascular aneurysms and vasospasm
	Cerebral angiography: detection of vascular aneurysms and vasospasm. Also, especially in posterior circulation, endovascular aneurysm coiling is effective
	?Swallowing studies
Special tests	VDRL, ?CSF analysis
Prophylaxis	?
Consults	Neurology, neurosurgery, ?rehabilitation, speech
Nursing	Seizure precaution I/O, stool guaiac, above the knee elastic stocking
	Elevate head of bed at 30–45 degrees, egg crate mattress
Avoid	?

(continued)

TABLE 7–6: Diagnosis: Subarachnoid Hemorrhage (Continued)
Management
1. Prevention of vasospasm: nimodipine, 60 mg q4h PO or via NG tube q4h (contraindication: hypotension; use lower dose in liver disease)
2. BP control: nitroprusside sodium, 0.1–0.5 mcg/kg/min (50 mg in 250 mL NS)
Labetalol: 10–40 mg IV q30min
3. Seizure prophylaxis (controversial): phenytoin, 15 mg/kg IV in NS (max: 50 mg/min), then 300 mg PO/IV (4–6 mg/kg/day)
4. Morphine: 1–4 mg IV q2–6h (avoid oversedation)
5. Docusate sodium, 100 mg PO qh, *or* bisacodyl, 10–15 mg PO qh

TABLE 7–7: Diagnosis: TIA	
Disposition	Unit
Monitor	Vitals
	Cardiac monitoring
	Neuro check qh
Diet	NPO except medication if gag reflex intact (start diet after swallowing studies)
Fluid	MIVF (preferably without glucose)
O_2	≥2 L O_2 via NC; keep O_2 saturation >92%
Activity	Bedrest
Dx studies	
Labs	Blood glucose, CBC with differential, BMP, LFT, PT/PTT/INR, stool guaiac, UA
	Fasting lipid profile, ?serum/urine toxicology screen
Radiology and cardiac studies	Noncontrast CT of head, CXR, ?MRI (see MRI Contraindications), ECG
	MRI (sensitive for ischemic, small stroke or stroke in brainstem)
	Carotid duplex US, cardiac echo, ?Holter, ?swallowing studies
Special tests	?ESR, ?VDRL, ?RPR, ?ANA, ?anticardiolipin antibodies
	?Lupus anticoagulant
	?Hemoglobin electrophoresis, ?coagulation panel, protein C and S
	If patient placed on Lovenox → ?check anti-factor Xa 4–6 hrs after first dose
Prophylaxis	DVT prophylaxis after ruling out intracerebral hemorrhage

(continued)

TABLE 7–7: Diagnosis: TIA (Continued)	
Consults	Neurology, rehabilitation, speech
Nursing	I/O, Foley catheter, stool guaiac, above-the-knee elastic stocking, aspiration precaution, elevation of head of bed at 30–45 degrees, egg crate mattress
Avoid	?
Management	

1. Start ASA, 325 mg PO daily, ± Plavix, 75 mg PO daily, if CT/MRI is negative for bleed (hemorrhagic stroke)

- Aggrenox, 1 tablet PO bid, has been shown to be more effective than ASA for prevention of CVA

- Alternative drug that can be used is ticlopidine, 250 mg bid, but the side effects are neutropenia, thrombocytopenia

2. Heparin and warfarin use in atherosclerosis TIA is controversial

3. Heparin and warfarin are indicated in patients with cardiogenic emboli from atrial fibrillation (keep INR = 2–3, 2.5–3.5 in mechanical valve) (see exclusion criteria below for starting patient on heparin and warfarin)

4. BP management: Lowering BP in acute cerebral infarction is contraindicated unless patient has the following:

- BP: systolic >230 or diastolic >120

- Hypertensive encephalopathy is present

- Vital organs are compromised

- Cerebral ischemia secondary to aortic dissection

5. Labetalol, 10 mg IV over 1–2 mins, then repeat every 10 mins as needed, to a total dose of 150 mg (DC if hypotension, bradycardia, or bronchial spasm). Alternative: nicardipine IV at 5 mg/hr; ↑ by 2.5 mg/hr q5–15min to max 15 mg/hr. (DC if hypotension, bradycardia)

6. Docusate sodium, 100 mg PO qh, *or* bisacodyl, 10–15 mg PO qh

7. Tylenol: 650 mg PO/PR q4–6h PRN for HA or temperature >38°C

(continued)

TABLE 7–7: Diagnosis: TIA (Continued)

8. Consider statin for cholesterol management and secondary stroke prevention; also ACE inhibitor, thiazide diuretic, or both for BP management and secondary stroke prevention

Note: Patient on Lovenox: may consider checking anti-factor Xa 4–6 hrs after the first dose

Heparin and Warfarin Exclusion Criteria in Patient with Stroke

1. CT/MRI scan shows: hemorrhage, tumor, abscess, epidural or subdural hematoma

2. Current bleeding

3. History of GI bleeding, bleeding tendencies

4. Large infarction noted on CT/MRI scan

5. Neurologic deterioration secondary to severe cerebral edema

6. Recent surgery past 14 days

7. Severe uncontrolled HTN (BP >185/110)

MRI Contraindications

Absolute contraindications	Relative contraindications
Electronically, magnetically, and mechanically activated implants:	Electronically, magnetically, and mechanically activated implants: other pacemakers, e.g.,
• Cardiac pacemakers	• For the carotid sinus
• Cardiac defibrillators	• Insulin pumps and nerve stimulators
• Ferromagnetic or electronically operated stapedial implants	• Lead wires or similar wires
• Aneurysm clips	• Carotid artery vascular clamp
• Metallic splinters in orbit	• Hemostatic CNS clips
	• Nonferromagnetic stapedial implants

(continued)

TABLE 7–7: Diagnosis: TIA (Continued)	
	• Cochlear implants
	• Implanted bone growth/fusion stimulator
	• Prosthetic heart valves (in high fields, if dehiscence is suspected)
	• Hemostatic clips (body)
	• CHF
	• Pregnancy (claustrophobia)

8
Pulmonology

TABLE 8–1: Diagnosis: Asthma	
Disposition	Medical floor/unit
Monitor	Vitals, pulse oximeter
	Respiratory monitoring: consider peak flow rate before and after bronchodilator treatment
Diet	Regular
Fluid	Heplock (flush every shift)
O_2	≥ 2 L O_2 via NC; keep O_2 saturation >92%
Activity	?Bedrest
Dx studies	
Labs	ABG, CBC with differential and eosinophil, BMP, sputum Gram stain and C&S
Radiology and cardiac studies	CXR, ECG
Special tests	Peak flow rate pre- and post-breathing treatment
	Pulmonary function test before and after bronchodilator prior to discharge
	?BNP if not sure whether it's CHF or asthma
Prophylaxis	Consider inhaled corticosteroids, DVT
Consults	?Pulmonary
Nursing	Pulse oximeter, peak flow, smoking cessation
Avoid	β-Blocker in exacerbations
Management	
1. β_2-agonist	
Mild to moderate	
Albuterol: 2.5 mg via nebulizer q20min or 6–12 puffs via MDI	

(continued)

TABLE 8–1: Diagnosis: Asthma (Continued)
Severe
Albuterol, 2.5–5 mg, with ipratropium, 0.5 mg via nebulizer
Albuterol: 10–15 mg nebulizer over 1 hr
Note: If patient develops tachycardia/palpitation/tremors → use levalbuterol (Xopenex), 0.63–1.25 mg q6–8h
2. Methylprednisolone, 2 mg/kg × 1 dose initially, then 1 mg/kg IV q6h, then change to PO prednisone, 1 mg/kg/24 hrs (give daily or divide bid) (max: 60 mg/24 hrs), then taper
or
3. Prednisolone: 1–2 mg/kg/24 hrs PO (give daily or divide bid) (max: 60 mg/24 hrs)
4. If all above fails → consider epinephrine, 0.3 mL of a 1:1,000 SQ q20min × 3 doses
Terbutaline: 0.25 mg SQ q6–8h
or
Terbutaline loading dose: 2–10 mcg/kg IV, then maintenance 0.08–6 mcg/kg/min
Consider aminophylline loading dose, 5–6 mg/kg IV; give over 20–30 mins, then maintenance dose
IV maintenance dose
1–10 yrs → 1 mg/kg/hr
10–16 yrs → 0.75–0.9 mg/kg/hr
>16 yrs → 0.7 mg/kg/hr
5. Ipratropium and albuterol (Combivent): 2–4 puffs qid
6. Fluticasone (Flovent): 88–220 mcg twice daily (max: 880 mcg twice daily)
7. Montelukast (Singulair): 5–10 mg PO qh
8. Salmeterol (Serevent): 2 puffs bid

(continued)

TABLE 8–1: Diagnosis: Asthma (Continued)
9. If infection suspected → consider using antibiotics
10. ?Pulmonary rehabilitation

TABLE 8–2: Diagnosis: COPD: Acute Exacerbation	
Disposition	Unit
Monitor	Vitals, pulse oximeter
	Respiratory monitoring: continuous O_2 saturation
Diet	Regular
Fluid	Heplock (flush every shift)
O_2	≤6 L to achieve O_2 saturation ≥90% (high oxygen content can suppress CO_2 drive)
Activity	?Bedrest
Dx studies	
Labs	CBC with differential, BMP, Mg, ABG, troponin I, ?blood C&S
	Sputum Gram stain and C&S, UA
Radiology and cardiac studies	CXR (PA and lateral), ECG, peak expiratory flow rate
Special tests	?α_1-Antitrypsin level
	?PFT with bronchodilator when stable
	Theophylline level if patient on theophylline
Prophylaxis	Consider inhaled corticosteroids, influenza (flu) and pneumococcal vaccine, DVT
Consults	Pulmonary, respiratory therapist (smoking cessation)
Nursing	Continuous O_2 saturation monitoring
Avoid	β-Blockers in acute settings
Management	See Management: COPD; also consider antibiotics

(continued)

TABLE 8–2: Diagnosis: COPD: Acute Exacerbation (Continued)

Global Initiative for Chronic Obstructive Lung Disease (GOLD) Criteria for Disease Severity in COPD Patient

0 (At risk)	• Normal spirometry
	• Chronic symptoms (cough, sputum)
I (Mild)	• Forced expiratory volume/forced vital capacity (FEV/FVC) <70%
	• FEV >80% ≥ predicted with or without symptoms
II (Moderate)	• FEV/FVC <70%
	• FEV <80% or >50% predicted with or without chronic symptoms
III (Severe)	• FEV/FVC <70%
	• FEV <50% or >30% predicted with or without chronic symptoms
IV (Very severe)	• FEV/FVC <70%
	• FEV <30% predicted

Treatment Modalities for Global Initiative for Chronic Obstructive Lung Disease (GOLD) Stages for Patient with COPD

GOLD stages	First line	Second line
0–I	• ?Risk factor avoidance	• ?Short-acting bronchodilator PRN
	1. Smoking cessation	
	2. Influenza vaccine	
II	• ?As stage I + add long-acting bronchodilators, preferably inhaled	• ?Pulmonary rehabilitation

(continued)

TABLE 8–2: Diagnosis: COPD: Acute Exacerbation (Continued)		
III	• ?As stage II + add long-acting inhaled corticosteroids	• ?Pulmonary rehabilitation
IV	• ?As stage III + add long-acting domiciliary oxygen	• ?If respiratory failure → surgery

Source: From NIH, Global Initiative for Chronic Obstructive Lung Disease.

Management: COPD

1. β_2-agonist

Mild to moderate

Albuterol: 2.5 mg via nebulizer q20min or 6–12 puffs via metered-dose inhaler

Severe

Albuterol, 2.5–5 mg with ipratropium, 0.5 mg via nebulizer

Albuterol, 10–15 mg nebulizer over 1 hr

Note: If patient develops tachycardia/palpitation/tremors → use Xopenex, 0.63–1.25 mg q6–8h

2. Methylprednisolone, 2 mg/kg × 1 dose initially, then 1 mg/kg IV q6h, then change to PO prednisone, 1 mg/kg/24 hrs (give daily or divide bid) (max: 60 mg/24 hrs), then taper

3. Prednisolone: 1–2 mg/kg/24 hrs PO (give daily or divide bid), max: 60 mg/24 hrs, then taper

4. Consider aminophylline loading dose, 5–6 mg/kg IV; give over 20–30 mins, then maintenance dose

IV maintenance dose

1–10 yrs → 1 mg/kg/hr

10–16 yrs → 0.75–0.9 mg/kg/hr

>16 yrs → 0.7 mg/kg/hr

(continued)

TABLE 8–2: Diagnosis: COPD: Acute Exacerbation (Continued)
5. Albuterol, metaproterenol, or terbutaline, 2–4 puffs q30–60min, then ↓ to 2–4 puffs q3–4h
6. Ipratropium: 4–6 puffs q4–6h
7. Flovent: 88–220 mcg twice daily (max: 880 mcg twice daily)
8. Serevent: 2 puffs bid
9. Guaifenesin: 100–400 mg PO q4–6h for cough and clearance of the secretion
10. Consider using antibiotics (see pneumonia protocols)
11. Chest physiotherapy (controversial)
Recommended Antibiotics in Acute Exacerbation of COPD
• Augmentin: 875 mg PO bid
• TMP/SMX DS: PO bid
• Amoxicillin: 500 mg PO bid
• Doxycycline: 100 mg PO bid
• Levofloxacin: 500 mg PO bid
• Ciprofloxacin: 500 mg PO bid
• Cefuroxime: 500 mg PO bid
• Cefprozil: 500 mg PO bid
• Cefpodoxime: 200 mg PO bid
• Loracarbef: 400 mg PO bid

TABLE 8–3: Diagnosis: PE	
Disposition	Unit
Monitor	Vitals
	Cardiac monitoring
	Neuromonitoring
Diet	Heart-healthy
Fluid	IV access
O$_2$	≥2 L O$_2$ via NC; keep O$_2$ saturation >92%
Activity	Bedrest
Dx studies	
Labs	CBC, BMP, Mg, PT/PTT/INR, ABG, troponin
Radiology and cardiac studies	CXR (PA and lateral), venous Doppler (lower extremity), ECG, spiral CT
	V-Q scan if contraindication to spiral CT or pregnancy, ?pulmonary angiography
	?Impedance plethysmography (lower extremity)
	?Quantitative D dimer in patient with low probability of having PE
Special tests	Protein C&S, antithrombin III, ?factor V Leiden, lupus anticoagulant
	?Fibrinogen, anticardiolipin antibodies, ?hypercoagulable panel, ANA
Prophylaxis	?
Consults	?Vascular surgery for ?inferior vena cava (IVC) filter, ?hematology/oncology, ?pulmonary

(continued)

TABLE 8–3: Diagnosis: PE (Continued)	
Nursing	Pulse oximeter, stool guaiac, SCD
Avoid	?
Management	See Management: PE

Wells' Criteria for PE (Modified)

	Score
Clinical symptoms of DVT	3
Other diagnosis less likely than PE	3
Heart rate >100	1.5
Immobilization or surgery in past 4 weeks	1.5
Previous DVT/PE	1.5
Hemoptysis	1
Malignancy	1

Score	Probability of patient having PE
<2	Low
2–6	Moderate
>6	High

Source: Reproduced from Dr. Philip Wells, M.D., Msc., with permission.

Management: PE

1. If hemodynamic instability or extensive DVT → consider pulmonary embolectomy or thrombolytics (tPA/streptokinase) (check fibrinogen before starting thrombolytics)

- tPA, 100 mg IV over 2 hrs → then heparin infusion, 15 units/kg/hr (keep PTT 1.5–2.0 control) or streptokinase, 250,000 units IV over 30 mins → then 100,000 units/hr × 24–72 hrs → then heparin infusion, 15 units/kg/hr (keep PTT 1.5–2.0 control)

(continued)

TABLE 8–3: Diagnosis: PE (Continued)
2. If hemodynamically stable
• Heparin: bolus 80 units/kg IV → then 18 units/kg/hr, √ PTT 6 hrs after starting infusion (keep PTT 1.5–2.0 control)
or
• Enoxaparin (Lovenox): 1 mg/kg SQ q12h or 1.5 mg/kg SQ daily
3. Start warfarin (Coumadin): 5–10 mg PO daily (maintain INR 2–3) when PTT becomes therapeutic
4. IVC filter (indicated in patient who has contraindication to anticoagulant or patients with recurrent PE or massive PE)
5. Pain management (see Chapter 12)
6. Ranitidine: 150 mg PO bid PRN

TABLE 8–4: Diagnosis: Tension Pneumothorax	
Disposition	Unit
Monitor	Vitals
	Cardiac monitoring
Diet	Regular
Fluid	Heplock (flush every shift)
O_2	100% O_2
Activity	Bedrest
Dx studies	
Labs	CBC with differential, ABG
Radiology and cardiac studies	Serial CXR (AP and lateral), ECG, ?CT of chest
Prophylaxis	?
Consults	Pulmonary, ?cardiothoracic surgery
Nursing	Continuous O_2 saturation
Avoid	?

Management

1. Insert 16- to 19-gauge cannula at second intercostal space and midclavicular line over superior aspect of the rib and attach three-way stopcock and 100-mL syringe followed by thoracostomy tube

2. Thoracotomy tube (16–22 French): insert at fourth, fifth, or sixth intercostal space at midaxillary line and connect underwater seal

3. Treat recurrent pneumothorax with pleurodesis

• Intrapleural doxycycline, 5 mg/kg in 50 mL NS; premedicate patient with a benzodiazepine and infuse lidocaine, 4 mg/kg in 50 mL NS intrapleurally before doxycycline

  or

• Intrapleural talc, 5 g in 250 mL NS (respiratory depression has been reported)

TABLE 8–5: Diagnosis: Pleural Effusion	
Disposition	Medical floor
Monitor	Vitals
	Cardiac monitoring
Diet	Regular
Fluid	Heplock (flush every shift)
O_2	≥2 L O_2 via NC; keep O_2 saturation >92%
Activity	Bedrest
Dx studies	
Labs	CBC with differential, BMP, calcium, Mg, LFT, amylase, lipase
	Rheumatoid factor, ANA, ESR
Radiology and cardiac studies	CXR (PA and lateral), thoracocentesis, spiral CT, bronchoscopy
Special tests	PT/PTT, pleural fluid analysis (see below)
	Suspicion of pancreatitis, esophageal rupture: amylase
	Chylous fluid: TG levels
	Cryptococcal and *Histoplasma* antigen
	Tumor markers: carcinoembryonic antigen; complement C3, C4; α_1-antitrypsin
	Suspicion of SLE: ANA
	Suspicion of TB: PPD, Serum QuantiFERON-TB Test and QuantiFERON-TB Gold Test
	QuantiFERON-TB Test for latent TB infection
Prophylaxis	DVT

(continued)

TABLE 8–5: Diagnosis: Pleural Effusion (Continued)	
Consults	Pulmonary
Nursing	Pulse oximeter, stool guaiac
Avoid	?
Management	Chest drain; perform pleurodesis in recurrent cases

Use any of the following when performing medical pleurodesis: tetracycline and bleomycin *or* doxycycline *or* minocycline *or* mepacrine

Pleural Fluid Analysis Orders			
Tube 1	**Tube 2**	**Tube 3**	**Tube 4**
LDH	Gram stain	Cell count	Cytology
Protein	C&S	Differential	pH
Glucose	Fungal C&S		Adenosine deaminase (TB)
Amylase	AFB		
TG			

(continued)

TABLE 8–5: Diagnosis: Pleural Effusion (Continued)

Pleural Fluid Analysis

Fluid	Transudate	Exudate	Transudate	Exudate
Protein	<3 g/dL	>3 g/dL	CHF	PE, pulmonary infarction
LDH	<200 U/L	>200 U/L	Cirrhosis	Infection/TB
Specific gravity	<1.016	>1.016	Nephrotic syndrome	Malignancy
Fluid:serum protein ratio	<0.5	>0.5	Hypoalbumin	Collagen vascular disease
			Glomerulonephritis	Esophageal rupture/trauma
Fluid:serum LDH ratio	<0.6	>0.6	Constrictive pericarditis	Hypothyroidism
			Atelectasis	Pancreatitis

Note

- The following exudates can present as transudates: malignancy, PE, sarcoid
- The following transudate can present as an exudate: CHF
- Hemothorax: pleural fluid hematocrit:serum hematocrit ratio → >0.5 (50%)
- Chylothorax: TG >110 mg/dL
- If pleural fluid pH <7. 2 → may have possible empyema

(continued)

TABLE 8–5: Diagnosis: Pleural Effusion (Continued)
Light's Criteria for Diagnosing Pleural Effusion Exudate (Yes to One Criterion Means It Is an Exudate), 98% Sensitive and 83% Specific
• Pleural total protein/serum total protein >0.5
• Pleural LDH/serum LDH >0.6
• Pleural LDH more than two-thirds of the upper limit of normal for serum LDH
Note: With patient suspected of transudate but meeting Light's criteria (e.g., CHF patient recently diuresed), subtract serum albumin from pleural albumin. If it is <1.2 mg/dL, then effusion is exudates.

Source: From Light RW, MacGregor MI, Luchsinger PC, et al. Pleural effusions: the diagnostic separation of transudates and exudates. *Ann Intern Med* 1972; 77:507–513, with permission.

TABLE 8–6: Diagnosis: Hemoptysis	
Disposition	Unit
Monitor	Vitals, check H&H q2–4h initially, then q4–8h
	Cardiac monitoring
Diet	NPO
Fluid	Initially resuscitate NS/LR (wide open to 125 mL/hr), then place on MIVF
	?Blood transfusion
O₂	≥2 L O₂ via NC; keep O₂ saturation >92%
Activity	Bedrest
Dx studies	
Labs	H&H q2–4h initially, then q4–8h, CBC, BMP, LFT, type and cross PRBC
	PT/PTT/INR, NG aspirate guaiac, fibrinogen, stool guaiac, PPD, ?BNP
	Sputum Gram stain and C&S sputum, AFB Cx, UA, 24-hr sputum production
Radiology and cardiac studies	EGD, CXR (PA and lateral), CT of chest
	Bronchoscopy when stable, bronchial arteriography
Special tests	Upper GI series with small bowel follow-through, ?colonoscopy, ?bronchoscopy
	?V/Q scan, ?AFB, ?sputum fungal and cytology, ?ABG
	?Anti–glomerular basement antibodies, ?rheumatoid factor, ?complement
	?ANCA, hemosiderin-laden macrophage

(continued)

TABLE 8–6: Diagnosis: Hemoptysis (Continued)	
Prophylaxis	PPI
Consults	Pulmonary, GI, thoracic surgery
Nursing	NG tube (patient with hematochezia to evaluate upper GI bleeding); monitor urine output
Avoid	Heparin, Coumadin, NSAIDs, ASA

Management

• Transfuse 2–4 units PBRC if profuse bleeding or low H&H

• Ranitidine, 50 mg IV q6–8h, or famotidine, 20 mg IV q12h, or pantoprazole (Protonix), 40 mg IV bid

• If high INR → vitamin K, 10 mg IV/SQ daily, and have FFP, 2–4 units, ready

• Variceal bleed

Octreotide IV bolus: 25–50 mcg followed by continuous IV infusion of 25–50 mcg/hr or

Vasopressin: 20 units IV over 20–30 mins, then 0.2–0.3 unit/min for 30 mins, then ↑ by 0.2 unit/min until bleeding stops or max: 0.9 unit/min

Nitroglycerin paste, 1 inch q6h off qh, or nitroglycerin, 10–30 mcg/min infusion (50 mg in 250 D_5W)

9
Rheumatology

TABLE 9–1: Diagnosis: Gout/Pseudogout	
Disposition	Medical floor
Monitor	Vitals
Diet	Low-purine diet
Fluid	Heplock (flush every shift)
O_2	PRN
Activity	Bedrest with BRP and OOB to chair
Dx studies	
Labs	Serum and urine uric acid level, CBC with differential, BMP, Mg, calcium, PO_4, TSH
	UA, urine R&M, 24-hr urine collection for uric acid, LFT, ESR
	Ferritin, iron, transferrin
Radiology and cardiac studies	X-ray of joint involved (may show subcortical bone cyst)
Special tests	Aspirated synovial fluid analysis: Gram stain, cell count, glucose, light and polarized micrography for crystals, protein, C&S, 24-hr urine for uric acid
	Gout = monosodium urate monohydrate, negative birefringent crystals (needle shape)
	Pseudogout = calcium pyrophosphate crystals, weakly positive birefringent polymorphic crystal (rhomboidal shape)
Prophylaxis	?
Consults	?Rheumatology, ?surgery
Nursing	Elevate joint involved if possible

(continued)

TABLE 9–1: Diagnosis: Gout/Pseudogout (Continued)	
Avoid	Purine-containing products: meats, beans, peas, spinach, ETOH, liver, sweetbreads, diuretics, ASA, pyrazinamide, ethambutol, cyclosporin A
Management	See below

Note: Urine uric acid <600 mg/24 hrs → considered undersecretor

Acute treatment options for gout and pseudogout

1. Indomethacin: 25–50 mg PO q6h × 2 days, then 50 mg tid × 2 days, then 25 mg tid *or*

2. Ketorolac (Toradol): 30–60 mg IM, then 15–30 mg IM q6h/10 mg PO tid–qid *or*

3. Ibuprofen: 800 mg, then 400–800 mg PO q4–6h *or*

   Note: Avoid NSAIDs in renal failure

4. Etoricoxib: 120 mg PO daily

5. Methylprednisolone, 125 mg IV × 1 dose, then prednisone, 40–60 mg PO daily × 5 days, then taper

   Note: High-dose prednisone is usually tapered after 2–3 days

6. Colchicine: 0.5–0.6 mg PO 2 tablets followed by 1 tablet qh until relief (max dose of 9.6 mg/24 hrs), then 0.5–0.6 PO daily–bid (not commonly used)

7. **Pain management is essential**

Chronic management of hyperuricemia

Overproducers: allopurinol, 300 mg PO daily, may ↑ to 100–300 mg bid–tid q2weeks (max: 3 g/day)

   (Side effects: rash, leukopenia, thrombocytopenia, diarrhea, drug fever)

(continued)

TABLE 9–1: Diagnosis: Gout/Pseudogout (Continued)
Underexcreters:
Probenecid: 250 mg PO bid, ↑ 500 mg bid after 1 week, then ↑ by 500 mg q4weeks
Sulfinpyrazone: 50 mg PO bid ↑ to 100–200 mg bid–tid q2weeks (max: 800 mg/day)
Note: Ineffective for chronic tophaceous gout

TABLE 9–2: Diagnosis: Giant Cell Arteritis (Temporal Arteritis)	
Disposition	Unit
Monitor	Vitals
	Neuromonitoring
Diet	Regular
Fluid	Heplock (flush every shift)
O$_2$	PRN
Activity	Bedrest
Dx studies	
Labs	CBC with differential, ESR, CRP, LFT, ?fibrinogen
Radiology and cardiac studies	?Temporal arteriography, ?color duplex ultrasonography of the temporal artery
	?Head CT/MRI
Special tests	Temporal artery biopsy
Prophylaxis	?
Consults	Rheumatology, surgery for biopsy
Nursing	?
Avoid	?
Management	
• Severe symptoms (e.g., vision loss): methylprednisolone, 250 mg IV q8h daily × 3–5 days	
• Mild symptoms: prednisone, 1 mg/kg PO daily, then taper	
• Consider using cyclosporine-azathioprine or cyclosporine-methotrexate combination as a steroid-sparing recipe for steroid-resistant cases (efficacy unproved)	
• Low-dose ASA may be useful	

(continued)

TABLE 9–2: Diagnosis: Giant Cell Arteritis (Temporal Arteritis) (Continued)

• Calcium and vitamin D supplement due to chronic use of steroid and risk of osteoporosis

Giant Cell Arteritis
History
• Headache
• Jaw/tongue claudication
• Arthralgia/arthritis
• Anorexia/weight loss
• Vision disturbance
• Myalgia
Physical examination
• Temporal artery tenderness, erythema, swollen, and warm
• Vision disturbance
• TIA/stroke
• Scalp tenderness

TABLE 9–3: Diagnosis: SLE	
Disposition	Medical floor
Monitor	Vitals
	?Neuromonitoring
Diet	No salt and low-psoralen diet
Fluid	Heplock (flush every shift)
O$_2$	PRN
Activity	Up ad lib, BRP, OOB to chair
Dx studies	
Labs	CBC with differential, BMP, Mg, PO$_4$, calcium, LFT, PT/PTT/INR, ESR, CRP, UA, ANA
Radiology and cardiac studies	CXR (PA and lateral), ECG
Special tests	Complement CH50, C3, C4, lupus erythematosus cell preparation, Coombs' test, lupus anticoagulant
	Anticardiolipin antibody, antinuclear cytoplasmic antibody, DNA binding
	Rheumatoid factor, 24-hr urine for CrCl and protein
	• If ANA positive → check anti-DS DNA, anti-Sm, anti-Ro, anti-La, anti-U1-RNP
	• If drug-induced SLE suspected → check antihistone antibody
Prophylaxis	Influenza (flu) and pneumococcal vaccine
Consults	Rheumatology

(continued)

TABLE 9–3: Diagnosis: SLE (Continued)	
Nursing	?
Avoid	Procainamide, quinidine
Management	See Management: SLE

Classification Criteria for SLE

At least four of the following 11 disorders must be present to diagnose patient with SLE:

• Malar rash

• Discoid rash

• Photosensitivity

• Oral ulcers

• Arthritis

• Serositis

• Renal disorder

• Neurologic disorder

• Hematologic disorder

• Immunologic disorder

• ANA

Source: Adapted from Tan EM, Cohen AS, Fries JF, et al. The 1982 revised criteria for classification of systemic lupus erythematosus. *Arthritis Rheum* 1982; 25:1271–1277, with permission.

Management: SLE

• Methylprednisolone, 500 mg IV q12h × 3–4 days, then prednisone, 50 mg PO daily

   or

• Prednisone: 80–100 mg PO daily ($\uparrow$ up to 300 mg/day)

   Maintenance dose: 10–20 mg PO daily/20–40 mg every other day

(continued)

TABLE 9–3: Diagnosis: SLE (Continued)
Mild disease associated with arthritis, dermatologic changes, and serositis
• Hydroxychloroquine: 200–600 mg PO daily
• Methotrexate
Arthritis, arthralgia, and myalgia
• Ibuprofen: 400 mg PO qid
• Indomethacin: 25–50 mg PO tid–qid
Mild nephritis
• Azathioprine (steroid-sparing agent)
Severe nephritis, vasculitis, or CNS disease
• Cyclophosphamide
Renal disease
• Cyclosporine
• Mycophenolate

10
Toxicology

TABLE 10–1: Diagnosis: Poisoning		
Life-threatening poisoning		
Hemodialysis can be useful with the following poisoning:		
• Ethylene glycol		• Salicylate
• Lithium		• Theophylline
• Methanol		
Charcoal hemoperfusion can be useful with the following poisoning:		
• Theophylline		• Salicylate
• Phenobarbital		• Paraquat
Activated charcoal is ineffective for the following:		
• ETOH		• Lithium
• Iron		• Absolute contraindications to charcoal is corrosives
Poisoning (general management)		
1. Stabilize patient (ABCs)		
2. Consider elective intubation in comatose patient		
3. Call poison control		
4. IVF if patient hypotensive		
5. Oxygen		
6. Thiamine		
7. Glucose		
8. Naloxone		
9. Monitor vital signs and mental status		
The following drug overdose requires level to determine severity of overdose and treatment options:		
• Acetaminophen	• Ethylene glycol	• Methanol
• Arsenic	• Iron	• Salicylate
• Carbon monoxide	• Lead	• Theophylline

(continued)

TABLE 10–1: Diagnosis: Poisoning (Continued)		
• Digoxin	• Lithium	
Poisoning toxidrome		
Stimulants	**Depressants**	
• Anticholinergics	• Antidepressants	
• Amphetamines	• Cholinergics	
• Cocaine	• Narcotics	
• Sedative withdrawal	• Sedatives	
Signs and symptoms		
• Agitation	• Miosis	
• Fever	• Mydriasis	
• Hyperreflexia	• Respiratory depression	
• HTN	• Seizure	
• Hyporeflexia	• Sweating	
• Lethargy leading to coma	• Tachycardia	

TABLE 10–2: Diagnosis: Acetaminophen Overdose	
Disposition	Unit
Monitor	Vitals
	Cardiac monitoring
	Electrolyte monitoring
	Neuromonitoring
Diet	NPO
Fluid	Heplock (flush every shift)
O$_2$	PRN
Activity	Bedrest
Dx studies	
Labs	Acetaminophen (Tylenol) level q4h until zero, PT/PTT/INR, BMP, calcium, Mg, PO$_4$, LFT
	Amylase, lipase, CBC, ammonia, lactic acid
Radiology and cardiac studies	CXR (PA and lateral), ECG
Special tests	Serum/urine toxicology screen, serum ASA, ETOH level
	?Charcoal hemoperfusion, ?hemodialysis
	Plot level on Rumack-Matthew nomogram to assess severity (see below)
Prophylaxis	?
Consults	Poison control, nephrology for charcoal hemoperfusion, ?psychiatry
Nursing	I/O, aspiration precautions, seizure precaution, suicide observation, pulse oximeter

(continued)

TABLE 10–2: Diagnosis: Acetaminophen Overdose (Continued)	
	NG tube with suction, gastric lavage
Avoid	Tylenol-containing products, liver-toxic agents (statins, anticonvulsants)
	Nephrotoxic agents (if acute renal failure), heparin, warfarin, ASA

Management

- Gastric lavage: if ingestion <1 hr, insert NG tube, lavage with 150–200 mL of NS (if <5 yrs: 10 mL/kg)

- Activated charcoal with recent ingestion (1 g/kg PO or NG q2–4h); remove charcoal via NG suction before administering *N*-acetylcysteine (NAC)

Indication of NAC administration

- Serum acetaminophen level greater than "hepatic toxicity" line of the Rumack-Matthew nomogram

- Single ingestion of >150 mg/kg (or 7.5 g in an adult) by history and for whom results of a serum level will not be available within 8 hrs from the time of ingestion

- Unknown time of ingestion and a serum acetaminophen level >10 mcg/mL

- Laboratory evidence of hepatotoxicity (from mildly elevated aminotransferases to fulminant hepatic failure) and history of excessive acetaminophen ingestion

NAC Dosing

- NAC using above nomogram (best if used within 8 hrs)

- Use NAC protocol for further management

  1. 72-hr U.S. Food and Drug Administration–approved protocol: PO only

  2. 48-hr IV bolus protocol

  3. 20-hr infusion protocol: IV

(continued)

TABLE 10–2: Diagnosis: Acetaminophen Overdose (Continued)	
72-hr NAC oral protocol	**20-hr NAC IV protocol**
140 mg/kg loading dose	150 mg/kg over 1 hr
70 mg/kg q4h × 68 hrs	50 mg/kg over 4 hrs or 12.5 mg/kg/hr × 4 hrs
48-hr NAC IV protocol	100 mg/kg over 16 hrs or 6.25 mg/kg/hr
140 mg/kg loading dose	
70 mg/kg q4h × 12 hrs	

• If INR >1.5 → vitamin K, 5 mg PO/IM/SQ; if unresponsive → consider FFP

• If INR >3 → consider FFP, 2–4 units

• If nausea → see Chapter 12

Source: From Prescott LF, Park J, Ballantyne A, Adriaenssensm P. Treatment of paracetamol with N-acetylcysteine. *Lancet* 1977;2:432–434, with permission; and Smilkstein MJ, Bronstein AC, Linden C, et al. Acetaminophen overdose: a 48-hour N-acetylcysteine treatment protocol. *Ann Emerg Med* 1991;20:1058–1063, with permission.

Management of Adverse Reaction to IV NAC

Reaction	Treatment for adult	Treatment for pediatric
Flushing	Continue NAC without treatment	Continue NAC without treatment
Urticaria	Diphenhydramine, 50 mg IV	1 mg/kg up to 50 mg
Angioedema	Discontinue (D/C) NAC → diphenhydramine, 50 mg IV, and restart NAC at slower rate in 1 hr if symptoms resolve	D/C NAC → diphenhydramine → 1 mg/kg up to 50 mg and restart NAC at slower rate in 1 hr if symptoms resolve

(continued)

TABLE 10–2: Diagnosis: Acetaminophen Overdose (Continued)		
Reaction	**Treatment for adult**	**Treatment for pediatric**
Wheezing or hypotension	D/C NAC → give supportive care	D/C NAC → give supportive care
	Diphenhydramine, 50 mg IV	Diphenhydramine, 1 mg/kg up to 50 mg
	Consider decreasing infusion rate	Consider decreasing infusion rate
	Consider ranitidine, 50 mg IV	Consider ranitidine IV, 1 mg/kg up to 50 mg
	Consider epinephrine (1:1,000), 0.3–0.5 mL SQ	Consider epinephrine (1:1,000), 0.1 mg/kg
	Consider fluids	Consider fluids
	Restart NAC IV at slower rate in 1 hr if symptoms resolve or change to oral	Restart NAC IV at slower rate in 1 hr if symptoms resolve or change to oral

Source: From Bailey B, McGuigan MA. Management of anaphylactoid reaction to IV N-acetylcysteine. *Ann Emerg Med* 1998;31:710–715, with permission.

(continued)

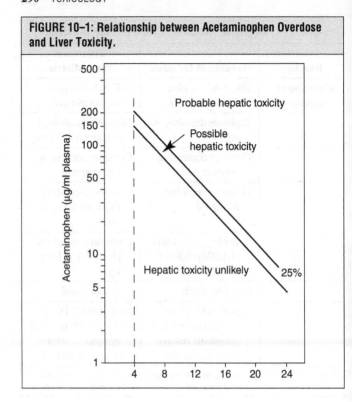

FIGURE 10–1: Relationship between Acetaminophen Overdose and Liver Toxicity.

TABLE 10–2: Diagnosis: Acetaminophen Overdose (Continued)

Signs and Symptoms: Acetaminophen Overdose (Toxic Dose: 7.5 g or >140 mg/kg)

Stage I (first 24 hrs)	Stage II (24–72 hrs)
• N/V	• ↑ LFT may be seen
• Diaphoresis	• Nephrotoxicity and pancreatitis may occur
• Pallor	• RUQ pain and tenderness
• Lethargy/malaise	• ↑ PT/INR, PTT, total bilirubin
• May be asymptomatic	• Oliguria, acute renal failure
• LFT may be normal	• ↑ Amylase and lipase
Stage III (72–96 hrs)	**Stage IV (4 days to 2 weeks)**
• ↑ LFT (LFT peaks during this period)	• Recovery slower in this phase
• Jaundice	• Labs may not normalize for several weeks
• Confusion (secondary to hepatic encephalopathy)	• ↑ LFT
• ↑ Ammonia	• Jaundice
• ↑ PT/INR, PTT, total bilirubin	• Confusion (secondary to hepatic encephalopathy)
• Hypoglycemia	• ↑ Ammonia
• Lactic acidosis	• ↑ PT/INR, PTT, total bilirubin
• Acute renal failure (secondary to acute tubular necrosis)	• Hypoglycemia
	• Lactic acidosis
	• Acute renal failure (secondary to acute tubular necrosis)

Note: Alcoholics, malnourished individuals, and patients on anticonvulsives are more prone to liver injury at low doses

TABLE 10–3: Diagnosis: ETOH Withdrawal	
Disposition	Unit/monitor bed
Monitor	Vitals
	Cardiac monitoring
	Electrolyte monitoring
Diet	NPO
Fluid	Fluid diuresis is essential (100–150 mL/hr)
	Note: Give thiamine before giving any glucose-containing solution
O_2	≥2 L O_2 via NC; keep O_2 saturation >92%
Activity	Bedrest
Dx studies	
Labs	CBC, BMP, calcium, LFT, PT/PTT/INR, Mg, PO_4, calcium, amylase, lipase, UA
Radiology and cardiac studies	CXR (PA and lateral), CT of head (if intracranial bleeding suspected from fall), ECG
Special tests	Serum/urine toxicology screen, ETOH level, vitamin B_{12} and folate levels
Consults	Social services, ETOH rehabilitation, ?psychiatry
Nursing	Seizure precaution, aspiration precaution, soft restraint PRN
Avoid	Carbamazepine, haloperidol (Haldol) (decreases seizure threshold)
Management	
1. Thiamine: 100 mg IV/IM, then 100 mg PO daily	
2. Folate: 1 mg PO daily	
3. Multivitamin: 1 amp IV, then 1 tablet daily	

(continued)

TABLE 10–3: Diagnosis: ETOH Withdrawal (Continued)
4. Tylenol: 650 mg PO q4–6h PRN for headache (caution in liver toxicity)
5. Withdrawal syndromes: lorazepam (Ativan), 1 mg PO/IV tid–qid; chlordiazepoxide, 50–100 mg PO/IV q6h
6. Delirium tremens: diazepam, 2–5 mg slow IV/IM q5min until patient calm, or diazepam, 5–20 mg IV q5–10min, then lorazepam, 2 mg PO q4h, *or* diazepam, 5–10 mg PO tid, *or* chlordiazepoxide, 50–100 mg PO/IV q4–6h
7. Seizure: thiamine, 100 mg IV plus $D_{50}W$ 50 mL IV, then lorazepam, 1–2 mg IV q5–10min × 2, diazepam, 5–20 mg IV q5–10min

Note
• If refractory to high-dose benzodiazepines → continue benzodiazepines and add phenobarbital, 130–260 IV q15–20min (get ready for intubation), or propofol, 1 mg/kg IV, induction agent for intubation
• Carbamazepine should be avoided in any withdrawal symptoms
• Lorazepam is minimally metabolized in liver (useful in patient with advanced cirrhosis)
• Phenothiazines, butyrophenones, and Haldol should be avoided because they ↓ seizure threshold

Symptoms: ETOH Withdrawal		
Time elapsed after last drink	**Clinical finding correlating with time elapsed after last drink**	
• 6–36 hrs	• Anxiety	• GI upset
	• Anorexia	• Headache
	• Diaphoresis	• Tremulousness
• 6–48 hrs	• Generalized tonic-clonic seizure	• Status epilepticus

(continued)

TABLE 10–3: Diagnosis: ETOH Withdrawal (Continued)		
• 12–48 hrs	• Hallucinations—visual (occasionally auditory or tactile)	
• 48–96 hrs	• Agitation	• Fever
	• Delirium	• HTN
	• Diaphoresis	• Tachycardia

ETOH level (mg/dL)		
>100 = intoxication	>200 = lethargic	>300 = coma

Clinical Institute Withdrawal Assessment for Alcohol Scale, Revised

Score	N/V	Headache	Paroxysmal sweats
0	No N/V	Not present	No sweat noted
1		Very mild	Barely perceptible
2		Mild	
3		Moderate	
4	Intermittent nausea with dry heaves	Moderately severe	Beads of sweat noted on forehead
5		Severe	
6		Very severe	
7	Constant N/V and dry heaves	Extremely severe	Drenching sweats

Score	Anxiety	Agitation	Tremor
0	No anxiety	No agitation	No tremor
1		More than normal activity	Tremor can be felt at fingertip

(continued)

	TABLE 10–3: Diagnosis: ETOH Withdrawal (Continued)		
Score	**Anxiety**	**Agitation**	**Tremor**
2			
3			
4	Moderately anxious	Moderate fidgety and restless	Moderate when hands are extended
5			
6			
7	Acute panic state/ delirium	Severely agitated	Severe when hands are extended

Score	**Auditory disturbance**	**Visual disturbance**	**Tactile disturbance**
0	Not present	Not present	Not present
1	Very mild harshness	Very mild photosensitivity	Very mild paresthesia
2	Mild harshness	Moderate photosensitivity	Mild paresthesia
3	Moderate harshness	Moderately severe photosensitivity	Moderate paresthesia
4	Moderately severe hallucination	Moderately severe hallucination	Moderately severe paresthesia
5	Severe hallucination	Severe hallucination	Severe hallucination
6	Extremely severe hallucination	Extremely severe hallucination	Extremely severe hallucination
7	Continuous hallucination	Continuous hallucination	Continuous hallucination

(continued)

| TABLE 10–3: Diagnosis: ETOH Withdrawal (Continued) ||
Score	Orientation and clouding of sensorium
0	Oriented and can do serial additions
1	Cannot do serial additions
2	Disoriented to date by ≤2 days
3	Disoriented to date by >2 days
4	Disoriented to place and/or person

Source: Reprinted from Sullivan JT, Sykora K, Schneiderman J, et al. Assessment of alcohol withdrawal: the revised Clinical Institute Withdrawal Assessment for Alcohol Scale (CIWA-Ar). *Br J Addict* 1989;84:1353, with permission.

ICU Admission Criteria

- Age >40
- Cardiac disease (CHF, arrhythmia, angina, recent MI)
- Hemodynamic instability
- Acid–base disturbance
- Electrolyte disturbance
- Respiratory insufficiency
- Infection (severe)
- GI condition (pancreatitis, bleed, peritonitis, hepatic insufficiency)
- Persistent temperature of >39°C (103°F)
- Rhabdomyolysis
- Renal insufficiency
- High dose of sedation requirement

TABLE 10–4: Diagnosis: Anticoagulant Overdose	
Disposition	Medical floor
Monitor	Vitals
	Cardiac monitoring
	Electrolyte monitoring
Diet	PRN
Fluid	Heplock (flush every shift)
O$_2$	PRN
Activity	Bedrest
Dx studies	
Labs	CBC, PT/PTT/INR
Radiology and cardiac studies	CXR (PA and lateral), ?CT of head to r/o intracranial bleeding
Special tests	?Fibrin split product, fibrinogen, ?serum/ urine toxicology screen
Prophylaxis	?
Consults	Poison control, ?toxicology
Nursing	Stool guaiac
Avoid	ASA, warfarin, heparin
Management	

- INR above therapeutic and <5 but no significant bleeding → hold warfarin

- ≥5 and <9 and no significant bleeding → hold warfarin

- ≥5 and <9 and high risk of bleeding → give vitamin K, ≤5 mg PO

  If rapid reversal needed → 2–4 mg PO and 1–2 mg after 24 hrs

- >9 and no significant bleeding → hold warfarin and give vitamin K, 5–10 mg PO

(continued)

TABLE 10–4: Diagnosis: Anticoagulant Overdose (Continued)
• Severe bleeding with any INR → hold warfarin and give vitamin K, 10 mg IV, slow infusion; supplement with FFP or prothrombin complex concentrate or recombinant factor VIIa depending on urgency; vitamin K, 10 mg IV slow infusion can be repeated q12h PRN
• Life-threatening bleeding with any INR → hold warfarin and give prothrombin complex concentrate plus vitamin K, 10 mg IV slow. Recombinant factor VIIa can be considered as alternative to prothrombin complex concentrate.

Source: From Ansell J, Hirsh J, Poller L, et al. The pharmacology and management of the vitamin K antagonists: the Seventh ACCP Conference on Antithrombotic and Thrombolytic Therapy. *Chest* 2004;126:204S–233S, with permission.

TABLE 10–5: Diagnosis: ASA (Salicylate) Overdose	
Disposition	Unit
Monitor	Vitals
	Cardiac monitoring
	Electrolyte monitoring
	Neuromonitoring
Diet	NPO
Fluid	MIVF (**Note:** Be cautious in cerebral and pulmonary edema)
O_2	≥ 2 L O_2 via NC; keep O_2 saturation >92%
Activity	Bedrest
Dx studies	
Labs	Serial salicylate level q2h, BMP, calcium, LFT, Mg, PO_4, CBC, PT/PTT/INR
	ABG, anion gap, lactic acid, ketones, DIC panel, UA
Radiology and cardiac studies	CXR (PA and lateral), ECG
Special tests	Serum/urine toxicology screen, serum acetaminophen
Prophylaxis	?
Consults	Poison control, nephrology, psychiatry, ?toxicology
Nursing	I/O, seizure precaution, aspiration precaution, suicide observation
Avoid	?
Management	See Management: ASA (Salicylate) Overdose

(continued)

TABLE 10–5: Diagnosis: ASA (Salicylate) Overdose (Continued)	
Signs and Symptoms: ASA (Salicylate) Overdose	
• Hyperventilation	• Respiratory arrest
• N/V	• Dehydration
• Pancreatitis	• GI perforation
• Altered mental status	• Tachypnea
• Agitation	• Noncardiogenic pulmonary edema
• Tinnitus	• Hypotension
• Deafness	• Hyperthermia
• Seizure	• Cerebral edema
• Disseminated intravascular coagulation	• Bleeding
• Initially respiratory alkalosis, then high anion gap metabolic acidosis	
Management: ASA (Salicylate) Overdose	
Less than 50 mg/dL (asymptomatic)	
51–110 mg/dL (mild to moderate toxicity)	
110–120 mg/dL (severe toxicity)	
• Activated charcoal (1 g/kg; max: up to 50 g PO) in water or sorbitol via NG tube	
• Alkalinize urine with NaHCO$_3$	
1. Give bolus of NaHCO$_3$, 2–3 mEq/kg IV push (adult dosage)	
2. Then give maintenance of 132 mEq NaHCO$_3$ in 1 L D$_5$W at 250 mL/hr (adult dose)	
3. For pediatric patient use 100 mEq NaHCO$_3$ in 1 L D$_5$W at 1.5–2.0 times maintenance	
Note: Do not use acetazolamide to alkalinize the urine	

(continued)

TABLE 10–5: Diagnosis: ASA (Salicylate) Overdose (Continued)

- Consider hemodialysis in following conditions:

  1. Profoundly altered mental status

  2. Pulmonary or cerebral edema

  3. Renal failure

  4. Salicylate level >100 mg/dL (7.2 mmol/L)

  5. Seizure

  6. Severe acidosis

  7. Fluid overload that prevents the administration of $NaHCO_3$

  8. Clinical deterioration despite aggressive and appropriate supportive care

TABLE 10–6: Diagnosis: Benzodiazepine Overdose	
Disposition	Unit
Monitor	Vitals: BP
	Cardiac monitoring
	Electrolyte monitoring (blood glucose)
	Respiration monitoring
	Neuromonitoring
Diet	NPO
Fluid	Heplock (flush every shift)
O$_2$	≥2 L O$_2$ via NC; keep O$_2$ saturation >92%
Activity	Bedrest
Dx studies	
Labs	BMP, calcium, Mg, PO$_4$, LFT
Radiology and cardiac studies	CXR (PA and lateral), ECG
Special tests	Serum/urine toxicology screen, serum acetaminophen and ASA, ETOH level
Prophylaxis	?
Consults	Poison control, ?psychiatry, ?toxicology
Nursing	Seizure precaution, aspiration precaution, suicide observation, oral airway at bedside
Avoid	**Note:** Avoid flumazenil in chronic benzodiazepine users and in mixed overdose. If used in these cases, flumazenil can precipitate seizure.
Management	
• Supportive care (respiratory support)	

(continued)

TABLE 10–6: Diagnosis: Benzodiazepine Overdose (Continued)

- May use activated charcoal in early presentation (50 g in water or sorbitol via NG tube)

- Flumazenil: 0.2 mg IV over 30 secs → 30 secs later → 0.3 mg IV over 30 secs → 30 secs later → 0.5 mg (max: 5 mg); use with caution in chronic benzodiazepine users

Signs and Symptoms: Benzodiazepine Poisoning	
• Blurred vision	• Irritability
• Confusion	• Lethargy leading to coma
• Dizziness	• Poor muscle tone
• Hallucinations	• Respiratory depression
• Hypothermia	• Slurred speech
• Psychomotor agitation, combative	• Delirium
• Autonomic instability	• Seizure
• Elevated BP	• Tachycardia

TABLE 10–7: Diagnosis: Carbon Monoxide Poisoning	
Disposition	Unit
Monitor	Vitals
	Cardiac monitoring
	Electrolyte monitoring
	Neuromonitoring
Diet	NPO
Fluid	Heplock (flush every shift)
O_2	100% O_2 via high-flow face mask
Activity	Bedrest
Dx studies	
Labs	CBC, ABG, BMP, calcium, Mg, PO_4, LFT, troponin q8h × 8, CPK-MB q6h × 3, UA
Radiology and cardiac studies	CXR (PA and lateral), ECG, head CT
Special tests	Carboxyhemoglobin level (arterial or venous sample is acceptable)
	Serum/urine toxicology screen, serum acetaminophen and ASA, lactic acid, ?ETOH level
Prophylaxis	?
Consults	Poison control, ?psychiatry, ?toxicology, social services
Nursing	Seizure precaution, aspiration precaution, suicide observation
Avoid	?
Management	See Management: Carbon Monoxide Poisoning

(continued)

TABLE 10–7: Diagnosis: Carbon Monoxide Poisoning (Continued)
Signs and Symptoms: Carbon Monoxide Poisoning
• Nausea
• Vomiting
• Headache
• Lethargy leading to coma
• Malaise
• Seizure
Management: Carbon Monoxide Poisoning
• Give 100% oxygen via high-flow face mask
• Continue 100% oxygen until carboxyhemoglobin level is <5–10%
• Consider hyperbaric oxygen if unconscious, cardiac dysfunction, acidosis, neurologic focus, or pregnancy

TABLE 10–8: Diagnosis: Cocaine Abuse	
Disposition	Unit
Monitor	Vitals
	Cardiac monitoring
	Electrolyte monitoring
	Neuromonitoring
Diet	NPO
Fluid	Heplock (flush every shift)
O₂	≥ 2 L O_2 via NC; keep O_2 saturation >92%
Activity	Bedrest
Dx studies	
Labs	CBC, BMP, Mg, PO_4, calcium, ABG (for withdrawal, decreased respiratory drive)
	Troponin q8h × 3, CPK-MB q6h × 4, LFT, UA and urine R&M
Radiology and cardiac studies	CXR (PA and lateral), ECG, CT of head if seizure occurs
Special tests	Serum/urine toxicology screen, ?HIV
Prophylaxis	?
Consults	?Psychiatry, social services, ?toxicology
Nursing	Seizure precaution, aspiration precaution
Avoid	Avoid nonselective β-blocker, succinylcholine
Management	
• Hyperthermia: cooling with ice water baths, mist and fans, and ice packs until a core temperature of 101–102°F is reached within 30–45 mins (avoid phenothiazines)	
• Seizure control: benzodiazepines	
• Sedation: benzodiazepines	

(continued)

TABLE 10–8: Diagnosis: Cocaine Abuse (Continued)
• Chest pain/MI: benzodiazepines, ASA and nitrates ± calcium channel blockers and α-blockers (phentolamine)
• HTN: nitroprusside, nitroglycerin, phentolamine, or hydralazine (use with pregnancy)
May use selective β-blocker (esmolol) but avoid nonselective due to its unopposed α activity
• Pneumothorax, hemothorax, and pneumomediastinum may be managed with tube thoracostomy, needle aspiration, or expectant management
• Tachyarrhythmias: calcium channel blocker and lidocaine (avoid nonselective β-blocker)
• Rhabdomyolysis: fluids and urine alkalization (mannitol and furosemide to have urine output of 3 mL/kg/hr)
Signs and Symptoms: Cocaine Overdose
• HTN
• CNS bleed
• Tachycardia
• MI, stroke
• Bowel infarction
• Rhabdomyolysis
• Hyperpyrexia
• Seizures
• Arrhythmia (ventricular tachycardia, ventricular fibrillation)
• Diaphoresis
• Euphoria
• Obstetric complication

(continued)

TABLE 10–8: Diagnosis: Cocaine Abuse (Continued)
Signs and Symptoms: Cocaine Withdrawal
• Dysphoria
• Increased appetite
• Hypersomnia, vivid dreams
• Lack of energy (fatigue)
• Intense craving for the drug
• Dysphoric mood

TABLE 10-9: Diagnosis: Digoxin Toxicity	
Disposition	Unit
Monitor	Vitals
	Cardiac monitoring
	Electrolyte monitoring, mainly K^+
Diet	NPO
Fluid	Heplock (flush every shift)
O_2	PRN
Activity	Bedrest
Dx studies	
Labs	Digoxin level, BMP, calcium, Mg, PO_4
Radiology and cardiac studies	CXR (PA and lateral), ECG
Special tests	?Serum/urine toxicology screen, ?serum acetaminophen and ASA
Prophylaxis	?
Consults	Poison control, cardiology, ?psychiatry, ?toxicology, ?social services
Nursing	Seizure precaution, aspiration precaution
Avoid	Calcium and potassium-containing products
Management	See Management: Digoxin Overdose
Signs and Symptoms: Digoxin Overdose	
• Arrhythmia	
• Abdominal pain	
• Blurred vision	
• Confusion/delirium	
• Color perception disturbance	
• Headache	

(continued)

TABLE 10–9: Diagnosis: Digoxin Toxicity (Continued)
• ↑ K⁺
• N/V
Management: Digoxin Overdose
• Perform GI decontamination if patient presents within 8 hrs of ingestion
• If serum K⁺ >5.5 mEq/L → see Table 6–4 (avoid calcium)
• Digibind [digoxin-specific Fab antibody fragments (DSAF)] indications:
• Ventricular arrhythmias
• Bradyarrhythmias unresponsive to atropine or pacemaker
• Ingestion of >10 mg of digoxin in adults or ≥4 mg in children
• Plasma digoxin concentration above 10 ng/mL (13 nmol/L)
• Serum K⁺ >5.5 mEq/L in addition to life-threatening arrhythmia
Administration of DSAF
1. The IV dose is given over 15–30 mins but can be given bolus in cardiac arrest
2. Dosing depends on steady-state serum digitalis concentration (SDC) or if total amount ingested is known
3. If total amount ingested is known, then follow
A. Total body load (TBL) = dose ingested (mg) for digitoxin (which has 100% bioavailability)
B. TBL = dose ingested (mg) × 0.8 for digoxin (which has 80% bioavailability)
C. Number of vials = TBL/0.6
4. If steady-state SDC is not known
A. Give 10 vials; repeat with another 10 vials if indicated
B. Chronic toxicity: give 6 vials to an adult; one vial to a child

(continued)

TABLE 10–9: Diagnosis: Digoxin Toxicity (Continued)

5. If the steady-state SDC is known

A. **TBL** = [SDC (mg) × 5.6 × weight (kg)]/1,000

B. **TBL** = [SDC (mg) × 0.56 × weight (kg)]/1,000

   (Digitoxin has a much smaller volume of distribution: approximately 0.56 L/kg)

C. **Calculation of the equimolar dose of DSAF**

   Molecular weight of DSAF: 50,000; molecular weight of digitoxin: 781

   I. Dose of DSAF (mg) = TBL × (50,000/781) = TBL × 64

   II. 1 vial of DSAF contains 40 mg, which neutralizes approximately 0.6 mg of digoxin (0.6 × 64 = 40).

   Thus, number of vials = TBL/0.6

   If we substitute this in equations A and B, where 0.6 divides roughly easily into the volumes of distribution for digoxin and digitoxin (5.6 and 0.56, respectively):

D. **Number of vials for digoxin** = [SDC × weight (kg)]/100

E. **Number of vials for digitoxin** = [SDC × weight (kg)]/1,000

Hemodialysis or hemoperfusion can help control hyperkalemia or volume overload

Source: From Antman EM, Wenger TL, Butler VP, et al. Treatment of 150 cases of life-threatening digitalis intoxication with digoxin-specific Fab antibody fragments. Final report of a multicenter study. *Circulation* 1990;81:1744, with permission.

TABLE 10–10: Diagnosis: Ethylene Glycol Overdose	
Disposition	Monitor bed/unit
Monitor	Vitals
	Cardiac monitoring
	Electrolyte monitoring
Diet	NPO
Fluid	Fluid diuresis essential
O_2	≥ 2 L O_2 via NC; keep O_2 saturation >92%
Activity	Bedrest
Dx studies	
Labs	UA, check urine for crystals, BMP, Mg, PO_4, calcium, serum osmolality
Radiology and cardiac studies	CXR (PA and lateral), ECG
Special tests	Serum/urine toxicology screen, serum acetaminophen and ASA, ETOH level
Prophylaxis	?
Consults	Poison control, nephrology, ?psychiatry, ?toxicology, social services
Nursing	I/O, seizure precaution, aspiration precaution, suicide observation
Avoid	?
Management	See Management: Ethylene Glycol Overdose
Signs and Symptoms: Ethylene Glycol Overdose	
• Lethargy leading to coma	
• Tachypnea	
• Flank pain	
• Renal failure (acute tubular necrosis)	

(continued)

TABLE 10–10: Diagnosis: Ethylene Glycol Overdose (Continued)
• Pulmonary edema
• Calcium oxalate crystals in urine
Management: Ethylene Glycol Overdose
• Supportive care
• Calculate osmolal gap
• Forced diuresis with IVF and mannitol: bolus: 0.5–1 g/kg, then
0.25–0.5 g/kg q4–6h; usual adult dose: 20–200 g/24 hrs
• Fomepizole (Antizol): loading dose of 15 mg/kg IV, then
10 mg/kg IV q12h for 4 doses, then 15 mg/kg IV q12h thereafter until ethylene glycol level is <20 mg/dL and patient is asymptomatic with normal pH
• Ethanol: initial dose: 600 mg/kg IV (equivalent to 7.6 mL/kg using a 10% solution), then
Nondrinker: 66 mg/kg/hr (equivalent to 0.83 mL/kg/hr using a 10% solution)
Chronic drinker: 154 mg/kg/hr (equivalent to 1.96 mL/kg/hr using a 10% solution)
• Dialysis if
Severe acidosis (**Note:** Continue ethanol during dialysis)
Renal failure
Ethylene glycol level of ≤50 mg/dL
• Folic acid: 50–70 mg IV q4h × day 1
• Thiamine: 100 mg IM q6h
• Pyridoxine: 50 mg IM q6h
• Charcoal is not effective

TABLE 10–11: Diagnosis: Iron Overdose	
Disposition	Medical floor
Monitor	Vitals
	Cardiac monitoring
	Neuromonitoring
Diet	NPO
Fluid	Heplock (flush every shift)
O_2	PRN
Activity	Bedrest
Dx studies	
Labs	CBC, BMP, calcium, Mg, PO_4, LFT, PT/INR/PTT, serum iron, TIBC, % saturation, TSH
	Type and cross PRBC
Radiology and cardiac studies	KUB (to determine tablets in intestine), ECG
Special tests	?Serum/urine toxicology screen, ?serum acetaminophen and ASA
Prophylaxis	?
Consults	Poison control, ?psychiatry, ?toxicology, ?social services
Nursing	I/O (maintain urine output >2 mL/kg/hr), seizure precaution, aspiration precaution
Avoid	?
Management	Whole-bowel irrigation is treatment of choice

(continued)

TABLE 10–11: Diagnosis: Iron Overdose (Continued)

If presentation ≤30 mins → induce emesis (charcoal is not effective)

- 6 mos–1 yr: Ipecac syrup, 5–10 mL PO followed by 10–20 mL/kg of water

- 1 yr–12 yrs: Ipecac syrup, 15 mL PO followed by 10–20 mL/kg of water

- ≥12 yrs: Ipecac syrup, 30 mL PO followed by 240 mL of water

- Can repeat dose one time if vomiting does not occur within 30 mins

If ≤20 mg/kg or unknown amount is ingested → consider gastric lavage

- Left side down with head slightly lower than body

- Place large-bore orogastric tube and check position by injecting air and auscultating

- Perform gastric lavage with NS 15 mL/kg boluses until clear (max: 400 mL)

If symptomatic or serum iron 350 mcg/dL

- Deferoxamine: 15 mg/kg/hr continuous infusion until serum level returns to normal range

If severely symptomatic or serum iron 1,000 mcg/dL

- Exchange transfusion

If hypotensive → place patient in Trendelenburg position and start IVF (10–20 mL/kg)

TABLE 10–12: Diagnosis: Lead Overdose	
Disposition	Medical floor
Monitor	Vitals
	Cardiac monitoring
Diet	Regular
Fluid	Heplock (flush every shift)
O$_2$	PRN
Activity	Up ad lib
Dx studies	
Labs	CBC, BMP, calcium, LFT, Mg, blood lead level, serum iron level
Radiology and cardiac studies	CXR (PA and lateral), ECG, ?x-ray fluorescence
Special tests	?Serum/urine toxicology screen, ?serum acetaminophen and ASA
	?Free erythrocyte protoporphyrin, peripheral smear, ?NCV
Prophylaxis	?
Consults	Poison control, ?toxicology, social services
Nursing	I/O, pulse oximeter, seizure precaution, aspiration precaution
Avoid	?
Management	
If blood level >70 mcg/dL and/or lead encephalopathy (treat for 5 days)	
• Edetate calcium disodium 50 mg/kg/24 hr continuous infusion: 1.0–1.5 g/m^2 or 250 mg/m^2/dose IM q4h	
• Dimercaprol (BAL): 4 mg/kg/dose IM q4h	

(continued)

TABLE 10–12: Diagnosis: Lead Overdose (Continued)
Symptomatic without encephalopathy (treat for 3–5 days)
• Edetate calcium disodium continuous infusion: 1 g/m^2 for 8–24 hrs or 167 mg/m^2/dose IM q4h
• BAL: 4 mg/kg/dose IM × 1 dose, then 3 mg/kg/dose IM q4h
Asymptomatic with blood level of 45–69 mcg/dL
• Edetate calcium disodium 25 mg/kg/24 hr: continuous infusion for 8–24 hrs or IV q12h
or
Succimer (Chemet): 10 mg/kg/dose PO q8h × 5 days followed by 10 mg/kg/dose PO q12h × 14 hrs

TABLE 10–13: Diagnosis: Methanol Overdose	
Disposition	?Monitor/?unit
Monitor	Vitals
	Cardiac monitoring
	Electrolyte monitoring
Diet	NPO
Fluid	Fluid diuresis is essential (100–200 mL/hr)
O₂	$\geq$2 L O$_2$ via NC; keep O$_2$ saturation >92%
Activity	Bedrest
Dx studies	
Labs	UA, check urine for crystals, BMP, calcium, Mg, PO$_4$, LFT, CBC, serum osmolality
Radiology and cardiac studies	CXR (PA and lateral), ECG
Special tests	Serum/urine toxicology screen, serum acetaminophen and ASA, ETOH level
Prophylaxis	?
Consults	Poison control, nephrology, ?psychiatry, ?toxicology, ?social services
Nursing	I/O, seizure precaution, aspiration precaution, suicide observation, ?social services
Avoid	?
Management	See Management: Methanol Overdose
Signs and Symptoms: Methanol Intoxication	
• Lethargy leading to coma	
• Blindness	
• CNS bleeding	
• Pancreatitis	

(continued)

TABLE 10–13: Diagnosis: Methanol Overdose (Continued)
Management: Methanol Overdose
• Supportive care
• Forced diuresis with IVF and mannitol: bolus: 0.5–1.0 g/kg, then 0.25–0.5 g/kg q4–6h; usual adult dose: 20–200 g/24 hrs
• Antizol: loading dose of 15 mg/kg IV, then 10 mg/kg IV q12h for 4 doses, then 15 mg/kg IV q12h thereafter until ethylene glycol level is <20 mg/dL and patient is asymptomatic with normal pH
• Ethanol: initial dose: 600 mg/kg IV (equivalent to 7.6 mL/kg using a 10% solution), then
Nondrinker: 66 mg/kg/hr (equivalent to 0.83 mL/kg/hr using a 10% solution)
Chronic drinker: 154 mg/kg/hr (equivalent to 1.96 mL/kg/hr using a 10% solution)
• Sodium bicarbonate
• Dialysis if
Severe acidosis (**Note:** Continue ethanol during dialysis)
Renal failure
Ethylene glycol level of ≤50 mg/dL
• Folic acid: 50–70 mg IV q4h day 1
• Thiamine: 100 mg IM q6h
• Pyridoxine: 50 mg IM q6h
• Charcoal is not effective

TABLE 10–14: Diagnosis: Opioid Intoxication (Heroin, Morphine, Meperidine, Fentanyl)	
Disposition	Unit
Monitor	Vitals
	Electrolyte monitoring
	Neuromonitoring
Diet	NPO
Fluid	Heplock (flush every shift)
O$_2$	≥2 L O$_2$ via NC; keep O$_2$ saturation >92% (monitor for respiratory depression)
Activity	Bedrest
Dx studies	
Labs	BMP, calcium, Mg, PO$_4$, LFT, CBC, ABG
Radiology and cardiac studies	CXR (PA and lateral), ECG
Special tests	Serum/urine toxicology screen, ?HIV
Prophylaxis	?
Consults	Poison control, ?psychiatry, ?toxicology, social services
Nursing	Seizure precaution, aspiration precaution
Avoid	?
Management	See Management: Opioid Intoxication (Heroin, Morphine, Meperidine, Fentanyl)
Signs and Symptoms: Opioid Intoxication (Heroin, Morphine, Meperidine, Fentanyl)	
• Abnormal mental status	
• Miosis (pupillary constriction)	
• Pulmonary edema	
• Anaphylaxis	

(continued)

TABLE 10–14: Diagnosis: Opioid Intoxication (Heroin, Morphine, Meperidine, Fentanyl) (Continued)

- Coma

- Hypotension and bradycardia

- Respiratory depression

- Acute respiratory acidosis

- Aspiration pneumonitis

Management: Opioid Intoxication (Heroin, Morphine, Meperidine, Fentanyl)

- Naloxone (Narcan): 0.4–0.8 mg IV (preferred), IM, intratracheal, SQ q2–3min as needed; may need to repeat doses q20min

Note

- If no response observed after 3 doses → question the diagnosis

- Use 0.1- to 0.2-mg increments in patients who are opioid-dependent and in postoperative patients to avoid large cardiovascular changes

- Duration of action of naloxone is 1–2 hrs

- Nalmefene: single SQ or IM dose of 1 mg may be effective in 5–15 mins (longer half-life than naloxone)

- IV: Green-labeled product (1,000 mcg/mL): initially, 0.5 mg/70 kg; may repeat with 1 mg/70 kg in 2–5 mins

- If opioid dependency suspected → administer a challenge dose of 0.1 mg/70 kg

- For postoperative opioid depression: blue-labeled product (100 mcg/mL): initial dose for non–opioid-dependent patient: 0.25 mcg/kg followed by 0.25 mcg/kg incremental doses at 2- to 5-min intervals

TABLE 10–15: Diagnosis: Opioid Withdrawal (Heroin, Morphine, Meperidine, Fentanyl)	
Disposition	Unit
Monitor	Vitals
	Cardiac monitoring
	Electrolyte monitoring
	Neuromonitoring
Diet	NPO
Fluid	Heplock (flush every shift)
O_2	≥2 L O_2 via NC; keep O_2 saturation >92%
Activity	Bedrest
Dx studies	
Labs	BMP, calcium, Mg, PO_4, LFT, CBC
Radiology and cardiac studies	CXR (PA and lateral), ECG
Special tests	Serum/urine toxicology screen, ?HIV
Prophylaxis	?
Consults	?Poison control, ?psychiatry
Nursing	Seizure precaution, aspiration precaution, ?toxicology, social services
Avoid	Pentazocine, nalbuphine, butorphanol
Management	See Management: Opioid Withdrawal (Heroin, Morphine, Meperidine, Fentanyl)
Signs and Symptoms: Opioid Withdrawal (Heroin, Morphine, Meperidine, Fentanyl)	
• Mydriasis (pupillary dilatation)	
• Piloerection	
• Yawning	
• Sneezing	

(continued)

TABLE 10–15: Diagnosis: Opioid Withdrawal (Heroin, Morphine, Meperidine, Fentanyl) (Continued)					
• Lacrimation, rhinorrhea					
• Anorexia					
• N/V and diarrhea					
• Anxiety					
Management: Opioid Withdrawal (Heroin, Morphine, Meperidine, Fentanyl)					
• Methadone: See table below to calculate dosing; avoid in severe liver disease					
• Buprenorphine: 0.1–0.4 mg IM; slow IV q6h					
• Clonidine: 1.2 mg/day in divided doses					
Methadone Dosing					
Signs and symptoms	0 Hrs	6 Hrs	12 Hrs	18 Hrs	24 Hrs
Mydriasis					
Rhinorrhea					
Lacrimation					
Goose flesh					
N/V					
Diarrhea					
Yawning					
Cramps					
Restlessness					
Voiced complaints					
Abnormal vital signs					
• 0 points if no symptoms present; 1 point if the symptom is present; and 2 points if the symptom is severe.					
• Give methadone, 1 mg, for each point.					

TABLE 10–16: Diagnosis: Organophosphate Intoxication	
Disposition	?Monitor/?unit
Monitor	Vitals, oxygen saturation
	Cardiac monitoring
	Neuromonitoring (CNS depression)
Diet	NPO
Fluid	Heplock (flush every shift)
O$_2$	100% O$_2$ (be ready for intubation in acute intoxication)
Activity	Bedrest
Dx studies	
Labs	BMP, calcium, Mg, PO$_4$, LFT, CBC
	RBC acetylcholinesterase (to confirm the diagnosis)
Radiology and cardiac studies	CXR (PA and lateral), ECG
Special tests	Serum/urine toxicology screen, serum acetaminophen and ASA
Prophylaxis	?
Consults	Poison control, ?pulmonary, ?psychiatry, ?toxicology, social services
Nursing	Foley catheter, seizure precaution, aspiration precaution, suicide observation
Avoid	?
Management	See Management: Organophosphate Intoxication
Signs and Symptoms: Organophosphate Intoxication	
First 24 hrs	
• CNS depression	• Hypersecretion

(continued)

TABLE 10–16: Diagnosis: Organophosphate Intoxication (Continued)	
• Cramps	• Lacrimation
• Weakness	• Salivation
• Muscle fasciculation	• Sweating
• Diarrhea	• Miosis
• Abdominal cramps	• Urinary incontinence
First 24–96 hrs	
• Respiratory and proximal muscle weakness	
Management: Organophosphate Intoxication	
• Decontaminate GI tract and skin	
• Airway management is essential	
• Atropine: 2–5 mg IV q15min until bronchial secretions and wheezing stop (may require >1 g)	
• Pralidoxime (2-PAM): 1–2 g IV over 30 mins or continuous infusion at 8 mg/kg/hr	
• Diazepam: 0.1–0.2 mg/kg IV; repeat if seizurelike activity	

TABLE 10–17: Diagnosis: Theophylline Overdose	
Disposition	Unit
Monitor	Vitals
	Cardiac monitoring
	Electrolyte monitoring
	Neuromonitoring: neuro check q1–4h
Diet	NPO
Fluid	Heplock (flush every shift)
O₂	PRN
Activity	Bedrest
Dx studies	
Labs	CBC, BMP, calcium, Mg, PO₄, LFT, PT/INR/PTT, theophylline level q6–8h, UA
Radiology and cardiac studies	CXR (PA and lateral), ECG
Special tests	?Serum/urine toxicology screen, ?serum acetaminophen and ASA
Prophylaxis	?
Consults	Poison control, ?psychiatry, ?toxicology
Nursing	I/O, seizure precaution, aspiration precaution
Avoid	?
Management	See Management: Theophylline Toxicity
Signs and Symptoms: Theophylline Toxicity	
• Seizure	
• Hyperthermia	
• Rhabdomyolysis	
• Tachyarrhythmia	
• Respiratory alkalosis	

(continued)

TABLE 10–17: Diagnosis: Theophylline Overdose (Continued)
• Hypokalemia
• Hypomagnesemia
• Hyperglycemia
• Hypophosphatemia
• Hypercalcemia
Management: Theophylline Toxicity
• Activated charcoal: 1 g/kg/dose (max: 50 g) PO/NG; give first dose with sorbitol; repeat one-half of initial dose q2–4h if indicated
• If >20 mg/kg ingested or symptomatic → consider gastric lavage
• Left side down with head slightly lower than body
• Place large-bore orogastric tube and check position by injecting air and auscultating
• Perform gastric lavage with NS, 15 mL/kg boluses, until clear (max: 400 mL)
• If serum level >60 mcg/mL or sign of neurotoxicity, seizure, coma, or life-threatening toxicity
• Consider hemoperfusion
• If seizure → Ativan, 1–2 mg/min IV

TABLE 10–18: Diagnosis: TCA Overdose	
Disposition	Unit
Monitor	Vitals
	Cardiac monitoring
	Neuromonitoring: neuro check q2–4h
Diet	NPO
Fluid	Diuresis is essential
O$_2$	≥2 L O$_2$ via NC; keep O$_2$ saturation >92%
Activity	Bedrest
Dx studies	
Labs	ABG, BMP, calcium, Mg, UA, CBC
Radiology and cardiac studies	CXR (PA and lateral), ECG
Special tests	Serum/urine toxicology screen, serum TCA level, acetaminophen and ASA
Prophylaxis	?
Consults	Poison control, cardiology, neurology, psychiatry, ?toxicology
Nursing	Seizure precaution, aspiration precaution, suicide observation, pulse oximeter
Avoid	?
Management	
• Lavage	
• Activated charcoal: 1 g/kg/dose (max: 50 g) PO/NG; give first dose with sorbitol; repeat one-half of initial dose q4h if indicated (continue until level drops to therapeutic range)	
• Magnesium citrate: 300 mL via NG tube × 1 dose	

(continued)

TABLE 10–18: Diagnosis: TCA Overdose (Continued)
• Monitor acid–base: keep pH at 7.5–7.55
• NaHCO$_3$ 50–100 mEq (1–2 amp) IV over 5–10 mins, then 100–150 mL/hr (2 amp in 1 L D$_5$W)
• If hypotension → IVF and pressors
• If seizure → benzodiazepines
• If conduction block → consider pacer
• If ventricular tachycardia or premature ventricular contractions → consider lidocaine or magnesium
• Indication for NaHCO$_3$
• Hypotension
• Arrhythmia
• Hemodynamic stable patient with QRS >100 msecs
• Seizures
Signs and Symptoms: TCA Overdose
• Coma
• Respiratory depression
• Seizure
• Hypotension
• Arrhythmia
• Cardiac conduction defect
• ECG changes
• Sinus tachycardia, ventricular tachycardia, premature ventricular contractions
• Prolonged QT, which can lead to torsades de pointes
• QRS >100 msecs
• ↑ PR interval

TABLE 10–19: Toxins and Antidotes	
Toxin	**Antidotes**
Acetaminophen	NAC
ETOH	Naloxone
Anticholinergic	Physostigmine
β-Blocker	Glucagon
Benzodiazepines	Flumazenil
Calcium channel blocker	Calcium
Carbon monoxide	100% oxygen, hyperbaric oxygen
Copper, arsenic, gold	Penicillamine
Cyanide	Sodium nitrate
	Sodium thiosulfate
Digitalis	Digoxin FAB
Ethylene glycol	Ethanol
Heparin	Protamine sulfate
Iron	Deferoxamine
Isoniazid	Pyridoxine
Methanol	Ethanol
Methemoglobin	Methylene blue
Narcotics	Naloxone/naltrexone
Nitrates	Methylene blue
Organophosphate	Atropine, pralidoxime
Phenothiazines	Benadryl
Warfarin	Vitamin K

11
Symptoms

TABLE 11–1: Diagnosis: Altered Mental Status	
Disposition	?Unit
Monitor	Vitals
	Neuromonitoring (if focal finding)
	Cardiac monitoring
	Electrolyte monitoring
Diet	?Regular/?NPO
Fluid	Heplock (flush every shift)
O_2	≥ 2 L O_2 via NC; keep O_2 saturation >92%
Activity	Quiet room, daily orientation, fall precaution
Dx studies	
Labs	CBC with differential, BMP, calcium, Mg, PO_4, vitamin B_{12}, folate, thiamine, LFT, TSH
	VDRL test/rapid plasma reagin, UA, troponin, ?ETOH level
Radiology and cardiac studies	CXR (PA and lateral), CT of head with and without contrast, abdominal flat-plate
	ECG, ?MRI
Special tests	?EEG, ammonia, ?ABG, ?serum/urine toxicology screen, ?UA C&S, blood C&S, ?LP
	?PTH, ?niacin
Prophylaxis	DVT
Consults	?Neurology
Nursing	Check mental status every day
Avoid	?
Management	See Management: Altered Mental Status

(continued)

TABLE 11–1: Diagnosis: Altered Mental Status (Continued)
Altered Mental Status
History
Baseline mental status
History of stroke or seizure
Risk factors of delirium
History of cardiac, renal, hepatic disease
History of psychiatric disorder
History of stroke
Poor nutrition
Dehydration
Multiple medication (polypharmacy)
ETOH dependence
Sedative dependence
Sleep disturbance
Recent surgery
Review medications
Physical examination **(perform complete physical examination)**
Monitor BP, pulse, respiratory rate, temperature
O$_2$ saturation
Observe general appearance
Look for signs of local and systemic infection
Mini-Mental State Examination
Look for signs of meningitis
Detailed neurologic examination
Look for signs of liver disease

(continued)

TABLE 11–1: Diagnosis: Altered Mental Status (Continued)	
Etiologies: Altered Mental Status	
Metabolic conditions	**Drugs**
Hepatic encephalopathy	Drug withdrawal: ETOH, benzodiazepines, barbiturates
Hypoglycemia/ hyperglycemia	
	Amphetamines/cocaine
Hypoxia/hypercarbia	Antihistamines: diphenhydramine (Benadryl)/hydroxyzine (Atarax)
Uremia	
Electrolyte disturbance	Narcotics: propoxyphene and acetaminophen (Darvocet)/ propoxyphene (Darvon)/ meperidine (Demerol)
Hyponatremia	
Hypercalcemia/ hypocalcemia	
Hypermagnesemia/ hypomagnesemia	Benzodiazepines: diazepam (Valium)/chlordiazepoxide (Librium)/flurazepam (Dalmane)
Acidosis	Steroids
Endocrinopathies	Anticholinergic drugs
Thyroid/parathyroid/ pituitary	Antiparkinsonian drugs
	TCA/phenothiazine/lithium
Vitamin deficiencies	Anticonvulsants: phenytoin/ phenobarbital/valproic acid
Vitamin B_{12}/folate/thiamine	
Toxins: carbon monoxide/ lead/mercury/manganese	Antimicrobials
	Third- and fourth-generation cephalosporins
Porphyria	
Infectious	Acyclovir, amphotericin B, quinines, isoniazid
Meningitis	
Encephalitis	Rifampin
Abscess	Cardiovascular drugs
Neurosyphilis	β-Blocker/digoxin/clonidine

(continued)

TABLE 11–1: Diagnosis: Altered Mental Status (Continued)

Infectious	Drugs
Systemic infection	Antineoplastic drugs
Bacteremia/sepsis	Immunosuppressive agents
Neurologic	**Miscellaneous**
Stroke/TIA	CHF and other cardiovascular causes
Seizure	Perioperative
Head trauma	Anesthesia/drug
Hypertensive encephalopathy	Anemia
	Embolism
Malignancy	Hypotension
Migraine	Fluid shift/electrolyte disturbance
Vasculitis	Dehydration
Limbic encephalitis	Sleep deprivation
	Depression

Management: Altered Mental Status

- Perform Mini-Mental State Examination

- Sitter

- Geri Chair

- Low bed

- Control noise stimulation

- Sleep management

- Reorientation

Treatment

- Thiamine: 100 mg IV or PO

(continued)

TABLE 11–1: Diagnosis: Altered Mental Status (Continued)

Use following modalities for safety and controlling agitation:

- Restraint (Posey vest, four-point restraint only in severe cases)

- Haloperidol (Haldol): 0.5–2 mg IV or 2–5 mg IM or 0.5–2 mg PO q30min (see max dose)

- Lorazepam (Ativan): 0.5–2 mg IV q6h 0.5–2 mg sublingual q30min (see max dose)

- Risperidone (Risperdal): 0.5–1 mg PO bid

- Olanzapine: 2.5–5 mg (Caution: may cause hyperglycemia and hypertriglyceridemia)

TABLE 11–2: Diagnosis: Anaphylaxis Reaction		
Disposition	?Unit/?monitor bed	
Monitor	Vitals	
	Cardiac monitoring	
	Electrolyte monitoring	
	Neuromonitoring	
Diet	Regular	
Fluid	Heplock (flush every shift)	
O_2	≥2 L O_2 via NC; keep O_2 saturation >92%	
Activity	Bedrest	
Dx studies		
Labs	CBC with differential	
Radiology and cardiac studies	CXR (PA and lateral)	
Special tests	?Mast cell tryptase (within 6 hrs of episode)	
	Intradermal testing and skin testing as an outpatient	
Prophylaxis	?	
Consults	Allergy immunology	
Nursing	Remove all old clothing	
Avoid	?	
Management		
Acute allergic reaction		
Medications	**Dose (adult)**	**Dose (pediatric)**
Benadryl	25–50 mg PO/IM/IV	1–2 mg/kg PO
Loratadine (Claritin)	10 mg PO	5 mg PO
Cetirizine (Zyrtec)	5–10 mg PO	2.5–5.0 mg PO
Prednisone	40–60 mg PO	1–2 mg/kg PO

(continued)

TABLE 11–2: Diagnosis: Anaphylaxis Reaction (Continued)		
Mild to moderate anaphylaxis		
Medications	**Dose (adult)**	**Dose (pediatric)**
Epinephrine 1/1,000 (1 mg/1 mL)	Epi Pen: 0.3 mg IM	Epi Pen Jr.: 0.15 mg IM
Benadryl	25–50 mg PO, IM, IV	1–2 mg/kg PO, IM, IV
Ranitidine (Zantac)	50 mg IV	1.0–1.5 mg IV
Cimetidine (Tagamet)	300 mg IV	5 mg/kg IV
Prednisone	40–60 mg PO	1–2 mg/kg PO
Methylprednisolone	125 mg IV/IM	1–2 mg/kg IV/IM
Severe anaphylaxis (treat as above plus add the following)		
Epinephrine		
1/10,000 (1 mg/10 mL)	0.005 mg/kg; give over 5 min (0.05 mL/kg IV in 10 mL NS)	0.01 mg/kg; give over 5 min (0.1 mL/kg IV in 10 mL NS)
1/100,000 (1 mg/100 mL)	0.75–1.5 mg/kg IV give slowly (1 mL/min)	
Source: From Gavalas M, Sadana A, Metcalf S. Guidelines for the management of anaphylaxis in the emergency department. *J Accid Emerg Med* 1998;15:96–98, with permission.		

TABLE 11–3: Diagnosis: Chest Pain	
Disposition	Monitor bed
Monitor	Vitals
	Cardiac monitoring
Diet	NPO except medication
Fluid	Heplock (flush every shift)
O_2	≥ 2 L O_2 via NC; keep O_2 saturation >92%
Activity	Strict bedrest with bedside commode
Dx studies	
Labs	Troponin q8h, CPK-MB q8h, BMP, calcium, Mg, LFT, CBC, PT/PTT
Radiology and cardiac studies	ECG, CXR (PA and lateral), ?ABG, ?CT of abdomen
	PE is suspected: spiral CT or V/Q scan, ?venous Doppler of lower extremities
	Aortic dissection suspected: CT of abdomen and chest, cardiac echocardiogram [TTE/TEE (preferred)]
Special tests	?Myoglobin q6h, lipid panel, TSH level, ?BNP, ?serum/urine toxicology screen
	Exercise stress test (see Chapter 1, Table 1–1), homocysteine level in young patient
	D-dimer if low risk for PE
Prophylaxis	?
Consults	?Cardiology, ?pulmonary
Nursing	Call physician if patient reports chest pain, stool guaiac

(continued)

TABLE 11–3: Diagnosis: Chest Pain (Continued)	
Avoid	Nitroglycerin in patient using sildenafil (Viagra), ASA and ACE inhibitors in pregnancy, caffeine-containing products; if renal insufficiency or pregnancy, avoid spiral CT
Management	Treat underlying cause; see below

• Assess patient: site/description/intensity (1–10)/radiation/ associated symptoms (N/V)

• Quick medical history (recent surgery, cardiac risks*)

• Assess for life-threatening conditions: MI/PE/aortic dissection/ tension pneumothorax/tachyarrhythmia

• Other conditions: GERD/esophageal spasm/herpes zoster/ costochondritis/anxiety

• If MI suspected → transfer patient to unit

　12-lead ECG (compare with previous ECG)

　0.4-mg sublingual nitroglycerin × 3 q5min (check BP before giving nitroglycerin); if chest pain continues and severe pain → consider morphine, 2–4 mg IV (**Note:** Hold nitroglycerin if systolic BP <90 or pulse <50)

　ASA: 325 mg crushed

　Troponin × 3 (first now and q8h), CPK-MB q8h × 24h

　If pain not relieved by nitroglycerin or morphine → consider Maalox, 30 mL, or GI cocktail

　If documented MI → see MI protocol in Chapter 1

• If GERD suspected → consider Maalox, 30 mL, or Pepto-Bismol, 30 mL

• If PE suspected → venous Doppler of lower extremity/?spiral CT/ ?V/Q scan/ABG

(continued)

TABLE 11–3: Diagnosis: Chest Pain (Continued)
• If pneumothorax suspected → get CXR (PA and lateral)
• Suspect aortic dissection: if back pain and ↑ BP → get abdominal CT

*Cardiac risks:** positive FHx, age, gender, DM, HTN, obesity, dyslipidemia, smoker.

TABLE 11–4: Diagnosis: SOB	
Disposition	Monitor bed/?unit
Monitor	Vitals, continuous O_2 saturation monitoring
	Cardiac monitoring
	Electrolyte monitoring
Diet	PRN
Fluid	Heplock (flush every shift)
O_2	≥ 2 L O_2 via NC; keep O_2 saturation >92%
Activity	Bedrest
Dx studies	
Labs	CBC with differential, CMP, ABG, troponin q8h × 3, CPK-MB q6h × 4, ?B-type natriuretic peptide
Radiology and cardiac studies	CXR (PA and lateral), ECG, ?spiral CT
Special tests	?Myoglobin stat and then q6h, ?serum/ urine toxicology screen, ?blood C&S, ?urine C&S
	?Carboxyhemoglobin, ?cardiac echo, ?PFT, ?methemoglobin
Prophylaxis	?
Consults	?Cardiology, ?pulmonary
Nursing	Stool guaiac
Avoid	?
Management	
Treat underlying cause	
1 L of NC can $\uparrow$ O_2 saturation by 3%, room air has 21% O_2	
• Assess for associated symptoms (think of the following: MI, PE, pneumothorax)	

(continued)

TABLE 11–4: Diagnosis: SOB (Continued)
• Medical history [e.g., COPD; **do not give high-flow O_2** (<2–5 L O_2)]
• Suspicion of possible CHF $\rightarrow$ give furosemide (Lasix), 40–60 mg IV (can be repeated)
• Suspicion of COPD $\rightarrow$ low-flow O_2 (max: 6 L O_2) $\rightarrow$ methylprednisolone (Solu-Medrol), 80–120 mg IV q6–8h
• Wheezing/rhonchi $\rightarrow$ breathing treatment [ipratropium and albuterol (DuoNeb)/albuterol]
• Suspect PE if recent history of surgery, oral contraceptive use, hypercoagulable state, immobilized
• Give 2 L O_2 $\rightarrow$ 4 L $\rightarrow$ 6 L and check O_2 saturation
• If patient doesn't respond to 6 L of O_2 $\rightarrow$ call respiratory
Give 40% Venti-Mask $\rightarrow$ check ABG in 30 mins
100% Nonrebreather mask $\rightarrow$ check ABG in 30 mins
BIPAP settings: ventilation/oxygenation (14/6) $\rightarrow$ check ABG in 30 mins
Do not leave patient with COPD on high-concentration O_2 for a long time; it can cause respiratory depression
Consider intubation
• **Note:** See Guide Tables for ventilator setting
• Sometimes albuterol breathing treatment can cause tachyarrhythmia $\rightarrow$ treat with levalbuterol (Xopenex), 0.6–1.25 mg q6–8h

Oxygenation Modalities and FiO_2 Relationship

NCO_2	FiO_2	Modality	FiO_2
1 L/min	25%	Venturi mask (Venti-Mask)	50%
2 L/min	29%	Simple O_2 mask	60%
3 L/min	33%	Partial rebreathing mask	75%
4 L/min	37%	Nonrebreathing mask	90%
5 L/min	41%		

(continued)

TABLE 11–4: Diagnosis: SOB (Continued)			
PaO_2 and saturation relationship			
PaO_2	30	60	75
Saturation	60%	90%	95%
Note			
• Venti-Mask is useful in patients who are CO_2 retainers; it provides precise administration of O_2			
• FiO_2 >60% for more than 3 days can lead to acute tracheobronchitis and diffuse alveolar damage			
• Oxygenation over 4 L $\rightarrow$ use humidifier			
• NC can support only 6 L of O_2			
• Oxygenation over 6 L $\rightarrow$ use high-flow NC			

TABLE 11–5: Diagnosis: Syncope	
Disposition	Monitor bed
Monitor	Vitals
	Cardiac monitoring
	Neuromonitoring
Diet	Regular
Fluid	IVF (if orthostatic or dehydration)
O$_2$	≥2 L O$_2$ via NC; keep O$_2$ saturation >92%
Activity	Bedrest
Dx studies	
Labs	CBC with differential, BMP, calcium, Mg, LFT, TSH, troponin level, UA
Radiology and cardiac studies	CXR (PA and lateral), CT/MRI of head, ?V/Q scan (PE), EEG, ECG, Holter, echocardiogram, carotid Doppler
Special tests	Check orthostatic BP, head-up tilt, ?urine C&S
	?Serum/urine toxicology screen, ?ABG, ?lipid profile, CPK level (rhabdomyolysis)
Prophylaxis	?
Consults	Cardiology, neurology
Nursing	Orthostatic BP, stool guaiac, TED stocking
Avoid	Antihypertensive medications, SSRI
Management	
BP and pulse (orthostasis) (orthostasis: ↑ in pulse of >10 bpm or ↓ 20 mm Hg systolic BP or ↓ 10 mm Hg diastolic BP when patient changes from recumbent to an erect position (usually occurs when 15–20% of fluid has been lost)	

(continued)

TABLE 11–5: Diagnosis: Syncope (Continued)	
Treat underlying cause	
• If vasovagal → high-salt diet (salt tablets, sports drinks) and volume repletion with NS	
• If orthostatic hypotension → consider fludrocortisone or midodrine	
• If ↑ heart rate → search for etiology	

Etiologies: Syncope (Loss of Consciousness for Brief Period)	
Neurally mediated	**Orthostatic**
Vasovagal	Drug-induced (see list below)
Carotid sinus syndrome	Autonomic nervous system failure: diabetes mellitus, ETOH, amyloid, parkinsonism
Situational (cough/ postmicturition)	
Cardiopulmonary conditions	**Cardiac arrhythmia**
MI	Sick sinus
Aortic dissection	AV block
Pericardial tamponade/disease	SVT/VT
PE	WPW syndrome/torsades de pointes
Aortic stenosis	**Neurologic**
Hypertrophic obstructive cardiomyopathy	TIA
Pulmonary HTN	Seizure
Medication-induced	Migraine
Diuretics/vasodilators	**Psychogenic**
QT-elongating drugs	Anxiety
Quinidine, procainamide, disopyramide	Hyperventilation

(continued)

TABLE 11–5: Diagnosis: Syncope (Continued)	
Sotalol, ibutilide, dofetilide, amiodarone	**Other**
Phenothiazines	Metabolic (glucose)
Amitriptyline, imipramine, ziprasidone (Geodon)	Anemia (bleed)
Erythromycin, pentamidine, fluconazole	ETOH use
Astemizole	Cataplexy
Droperidol	Acute hypoxemia

12
Symptom Management

TABLE 12–1: Agitation/Anxiety (Behavioral Management)
• Assess patient and check vitals
• Check medication list and electrolytes
• R/o delirium (see Table 12–6)
• Haloperidol (Haldol)*: 0.5–2.0 mg IV q30min or 2–5 mg IM or 0.5–2.0 mg PO q4–6h PRN (use with caution in elderly) *or*
• Lorazepam (Ativan): 0.5–2.0 mg IV/IM/PO q6–8h PRN (antidote: flumazenil, 0.2 mg IV/30 secs) *or*
• Hydroxyzine (Vistaril, Atarax): 50–100 mg IM/PO q6–24h PRN (avoid in elderly) *or*
• Droperidol: 0.625–2.5 mg IV or 2.5–10.0 mg IM (may cause QT prolongation) *or*
• Risperidone: 0.5–2.0 mg PO and IM (prolong sedation) *or*
• Temazepam (Restoril): 7.5–30.0 mg PO qhs PRN, long half-life (antidote: flumazenil, 0.2 mg IV over 30 secs) *or*
• Olanzapine (Zyprexa): 2.5–10.0 mg PO (prolong sedation; caution in patient with DM due to risk of hyperglycemia) *or*
• Ziprasidone (Geodon): 10–20 mg IM (as effective as Haldol; prolong sedation) *or*
• Quetiapine (Seroquel): 25–100 mg PO (may cause hypotension, prolong sedation)
• Consider Posey vest and/or four-point restraints to prevent injury to self and others
*Haldol: Start lowest dose in elderly and have naloxone (Narcan), 0.4–2.0 mg q2–3min at bedside due to respiratory depression.

TABLE 12–2: Chest Congestion
• Guaifenesin/potassium guaiacolsulfonate (Humibid LA): 1–2 tablets q12h, 600–1,200 mg q12h *or*
• Guaifenesin: 100–400 mg PO q4h or 600–1,200 mg PO q12h *or*
• Pseudoephedrine: 60 mg PO q4h
• Chest PT (flutter)

TABLE 12–3: Cough/Throat Irritation

- Guaifenesin (Robitussin)/brompheniramine and pseudoephedrine (Dimetapp), 10 mL q4h PRN; if congestion → Robitussin DM, 10 mL q4h PRN *or*

- Benzonatate (Tessalon perles): 100–200 mg PO tid *or*

- Menthol (Cepacol Lozenges/Spray) PRN (also comes in sugar-free; good for diabetics) *or*

- Menthol/benzocaine (Chloraseptic Lozenges) PRN

Note: Avoid Robitussin/Dimetapp in patients with HTN

TABLE 12–4: Constipation Management

Note: Maintenance management may require more than one class of drugs

Bulk laxative

• Psyllium (Metamucil, Perdiem, Fiberall)

• Methylcellulose (Citrucel)

• Polycarbophil (FiberCon, Equalactin, Konsyl Fiber)

  Examples

  • Bran powder: 1–4 tablespoon bid; onset >24 hrs

  • Psyllium: 1 tsp daily–bid; onset >24 hrs

  • Methylcellulose: 1 tsp daily–bid; onset >24 hrs

Osmotic laxative

• Magnesium hydroxide (Milk of Magnesia)

• Magnesium citrate (Evac-Q-Mag)

• Sodium phosphate (Fleet enema, Fleet Phospho-Soda, Visicol)

  Examples

  • Mg hydroxide/Mg sulfate: 20–30 mL daily–bid; onset 3–12 hrs

  • Sodium phosphate: 45 mL in 12 ounces of water; may repeat in 10 hrs, before colonoscopy; onset 1–6 hrs

Poorly absorbed sugar

• Lactulose (Cephulac, Chronulac, Duphalac)

• Sorbitol (Cytosol)

• Mannitol

• Polyethylene glycol and electrolytes (Colyte, GoLYTELY, NuLYTELY)

• Polyethylene glycol (MiraLax)

  Examples

  • Sorbitol 70%: 30–60 mL daily–tid; onset 24–48 hrs

  • Lactulose: 30–60 mL daily–tid; onset 24–48 hrs

(continued)

TABLE 12–4: Constipation Management (Continued)
• Polyethylene glycol: 4 L PO; administer over 2–4 hrs; useful before colonoscopy; onset <4 hrs
Stimulant laxative
• Cascara sagrada (Colamin, Sagrada Lax)
• Castor oil (Purge, Neoloid, Emulsoil)
• Bisacodyl (Dulcolax, Correctol)
• Sodium picosulfate (Lubrilax, Sur-lax)
• Docusate sodium (Colace, Regulax SS, Surfax)
• Mineral oil (Fleet mineral oil)
Examples
• Bisacodyl: 5–15 mg PO; onset 6–8 hrs
• Bisacodyl: 10 mg PR; onset 1 hr
• Cascara: 4–8 mL/2 tablets; onset 8–12 hrs
• Senna: 5–15 mg (max: 3 × daily) (useful in constipation due to narcotic use; onset 8–12 hrs)
Rectal enema/suppository
• Phosphate enema (Fleet enema)
• Mineral oil retention enema (Fleet mineral oil enema)
• Tap water enema
• Soapsuds enema
• Glycerin bisacodyl suppository
Examples
• Tap water enema: 500 mL PR until clear; onset 5–15 mins
• Phosphate enema: 120 mL PR; onset 5–15 mins (useful for acute constipation)
• Soapsuds enema: up to 1,500 mL PR; onset 5–15 mins (can cause mucosal damage)

(continued)

TABLE 12–4: Constipation Management (Continued)
Cholinergic agent
• Bethanechol (Urecholine)
• Colchicine (Colsalide)
• Misoprostol (Cytotec)
Prokinetic agent
• Cisapride (Propulsid)*
• Tegaserod (Zelnorm)
*This drug is available only through a limited-access program (by Janssen Pharmaceuticals and the U.S. Food and Drug Administration).

TABLE 12–5: Death (Pronouncing Death)
• When called to pronounce death, check the following:
1. Respiration (should be absent)
2. Pulse (should be absent)
3. Pupillary reaction (should be fixed and dilated)
4. Reaction to pain stimuli → sternal rub (should be absent)
• Document above being absent/present as well as date and time of examination
• Inform family member and primary care physician about the death
• Notify family member and ask family about having an autopsy performed
• Document probable cause of death
• Inform coroner if necessary
• Sign a death certificate
Death Note: Time and Date
• Patient name and medical record number
• Admission date
• Today's date
• Time you were notified by a nurse.
• Time the patient was seen by you.
• Document the following being absent on examination:
1. Respiration (should be absent)
2. Pulse (should be absent)
3. Pupillary reaction (should be fixed and dilated)
4. Reaction to pain stimuli: test with sternal rub or pressing on nail bed with metal (should be absent)
• Time the patient was pronounced dead, also document the date
• Document probable cause of death.

(continued)

TABLE 12–5: Death (Pronouncing Death) (Continued)
• Document whether the patient's family was notified about having an autopsy performed.
• Document that next of kin was notified.
• Inform coroner (if required)
• Document that the family member and primary care physician were notified
• Your name and pager number

TABLE 12–6: Delirium		
Assess patient		
Check vitals (BP, pulse, respiration, temperature), O_2 saturation, and I/O		
Check medications (examples of medications that can cause delirium)		
• Atarax	• Propoxyphene and acetaminophen (Darvocet)	• Chlordiazepoxide (Librium)
• Diphenhydramine (Benadryl)	• Propoxyphene (Darvon)	• Diazepam (Valium)
• Flurazepam (Dalmane)	• Meperidine (Demerol)	• Vistaril
Check labs		
• CBC	• Troponin I	• ECG
• CMP	• UA	• ?CXR
• BGM	• Toxicology screen	• ?Urine C&S
Management		
1. Sitter		
2. Geri Chair		
3. Low bed		
4. Environmental changes		
• Keep windows open at day time for sunlight exposure		
• Keep a clock and a calendar in the room for orientation		
• Make sure patient wears glasses and hearing aids while awake		
5. Make sure patient is well hydrated (be cautious in heart failure patients)		
6. Restraint (Posey vest, four-point in extreme cases)		
7. May consider sedation at evening to prevent "sundowning"		

(continued)

TABLE 12–6: Delirium (Continued)
8. Haldol: 0.5–2.0 mg IV q30min or 2–5 mg IM or 0.5–2.0 mg PO *or*
9. Ativan: 0.5–2.0 mg PO sublingual q30min *or*
10. Olanzapine: 2.5–5.0 (max: 15 mg/day) PO daily *or*
11. Risperidone: 0.5 mg PO bid (max: 6 mg/day in elderly); may cause hypotension *or*
12. Quetiapine: 25 mg PO bid (max: 800 mg/day) *or*
13. Clozapine: 12.5 mg PO bid (max: 450 mg/day); may cause agranulocytosis *or*
14. Ziprasidone: 20 mg PO bid (max: 80 mg/day) or 10–20 mg IM bid (max: 40 mg/day)

TABLE 12–7: Diarrhea

- If etiology infectious → check stool leukocytes, ova, parasite, and culture, CBC with differential, HepA, IgM, and IgG

- If etiology antibiotic-induced → check stool for *Clostridium difficile* toxin A and B

- Fluid replacement

- Search etiology of diarrhea before starting antidiarrheal agents

- Bismuth subsalicylate (Kaopectate): 1,200–1,500 mg PO after loose bowel movement *or*

- Loperamide (Imodium): 2 capsules PO initially *or*

- Diphenoxylate and atropine (Lomotil): 2 tablets or 10 mL PO qid *or*

- Metamucil: 1–2 tablets with juice *or*

- Sucralfate (Carafate): 1 g PO 1 hr before meal and qhs

Note: If *C. difficile* suspected → start patient on treatment before receiving toxin results and place patient under isolation precautions

TABLE 12–8: Dizziness
• Assess patient and check vitals
• BGM → low (50–60) → give orange juice → if <50 → 1 amp of glucose $D_{50}W$ (1 amp of $D_{50}W$ can ↑ glucose by 100)
• Check medications
• BP and pulse (check orthostasis)
[Orthostasis: ↑ in pulse of >10 bpm or ↓ 20 mm Hg SBP or ↓ 10 mm Hg diastolic BP when patient changes from recumbent to an erect position (usually occurs when 15–20% of fluid has been lost)]
• Perform fecal occult blood test to r/o GI bleed
• Check 12-lead ECG to r/o arrhythmia
• Check electrolytes
• Studies to consider: echocardiogram, Holter monitor, tilt table, CT/MRI, carotid Doppler tilt table

TABLE 12–9: Dry Nose
• OCEAN nasal spray *or*
• Saline nasal spray

TABLE 12–10: Dyspepsia/Heartburn

- Aluminum hydroxide, magnesium hydroxide, and simethicone (Maalox), 30 mL PO, *or* bismuth subsalicylate (Pepto-Bismol), 30 mL, *or* aluminum hydroxide, magnesium hydroxide, and simethicone (Mylanta), 30 mL PO, *or* aluminum hydroxide (Amphojel), 30 mL PO

- Omeprazole (Prilosec), 20 mg PO daily (PPI), *or* pantoprazole (Protonix), 40 mg PO daily (PPI), *or* H_2 blocker *or*

- Metoclopramide (Reglan), 10 mg 30 mins before meal *or*

- GI cocktail: Maalox *or* Mylanta, 30 mL; plus viscous lidocaine (2%), 10 mL; plus atropine, hyoscyamine, phenobarbital, and scopolamine (Donnatal), 10 mL

- Consider GI evaluation

TABLE 12–11: End of Life (Management of Patient with Dyspnea)		
Mild	**Severe**	**Critically Ill**
• Hydrocodone: 5 mg q4h *or*	• Morphine: 5–15 mg q4h *or*	• Morphine or fentanyl infusion
• Codeine: 30 mg q4h; can be given q2h for breakthrough doses	• Oxycodone and ASA (Percodan): 5–10 mg q4h	

Source: From *J Am Coll Surg* 2002;V194:381, Mosenthal AC, © American College of Surgeons, with permission.

TABLE 12–12: Epistaxis
• Assess patient and check vitals
• Have patient lean forward to avoid swallowing blood
• Apply pressure to distal part of nose
• Evaluate for anterior versus posterior
• Posterior bleed may require ear, nose, and throat (ENT) evaluation/consult
• Next step → chemical cautery: silver nitrate, trichloroacetic acid
• Next step → nasal packing
• Next step → Epistat catheter
• Next step → Epistat II catheter
• Next step → Merocel nasal tampon
• Check CBC with differential and PT/PTT

TABLE 12–13: Fall
• Assess patient and check vitals
• Stabilize patient (ABCs) and assess patient for injury
• Check medication list (also check list of medications that cause delirium)
• Ask current symptoms (dizziness, lightheadedness, headache, weakness)
• Search for etiology and treat appropriately
• Consider restraint chemical or physical restraint (Haldol, Posey vest)
Note: Also see Agitation, Table 12–1, and Delirium, Table 12–6

TABLE 12–14: Fever (Temperature >100.4°F)

- If first episode → investigate etiology

- Consider acetaminophen (Tylenol): one 650 mg tablet PO immediately

- Consider cooling blanket; discontinue when temperature ≤102.5°F

- Assess for phlebitis in patients with Foley, IV and arterial lines, decubitus ulcer, skin breakdown, rash

- Check previous CBC, CXR, cultures

- If suspicion of sepsis

    → Order CBC with differential, UA, urine R&M, urine C&S

    → Stool C&S, blood C&S × 2 15 mins apart from two different sites, stool *C. difficile* toxin A and B

    → Also consider CXR (AP and lateral), sputum C&S, and acid-fast stain

TABLE 12–15: Glucose (High)	
• Assess patient and check vitals	
• Check medication list	
• Give insulin according to sliding scale	
Note: Insulin sliding scale may vary from institution to institution	
• Check patient's last insulin/antihyperglycemic medication/other medications	
• Check for patient's diet status	
• Search for etiology: medications (e.g., steroids)	
• Blood sugar	**SQ** regular insulin to be given (units)
150–200	2
201–250	4
251–300	6
301–350	8
351–400	10
401–450	12
• Above insulin sliding scale varies from institution to institution	
• If >400 → check urine ketones, serum ketone, and BMP (serum ketone measures only acetoacetate)	
Check for serum β-hydroxybutyrate	
• Recheck blood sugar in 45 mins to 1 hr after giving insulin	
Note: See Chapter 2 for types of insulin regimens	

TABLE 12–16: Glucose (Low)
• Assess patient and check vitals
• Check for symptoms (sweating, tachycardia, dizziness, weakness)
• If between 50–60 → give orange juice with crackers
• If symptomatic or <50 → 1 amp of glucose $D_{50}W$ (1 amp can ↑ glucose by 100)
• If no IV access → glucagon 1 mg IM (side effects: N/V)
• Check blood sugar q30min to every hr until stable

TABLE 12–17: Headache
• Assess patient and check vitals
• Check medications (nitroglycerin)
• Recent procedure (spinal tap, epidural)
• Check for focal neurologic deficits
• Consider CT or MRI of head if intracerebral pathology suspected
• Treatment: low-flow O_2
1. Tylenol: 650 mg PO (check LFT; if high, consider alternative) *or*
2. NSAIDs: ibuprofen, 600 mg PO (check LFT; if high, consider alternative)
3. Antiemetics
4. Narcotics (if no response to above modalities)
5. Triptans or ergots for migraine headache (be cautious in setting of HTN)

TABLE 12–18: Hiccups
• Assess patient and check vitals
• Baclofen: 10–20 mg IV q8h first line
• Chlorpromazine (Thorazine): 25–50 mg PO/IM q6h second line
• Metoclopramide: 5–10 mg q6–8h second line
• Promethazine (Phenergan): 10 mg PO q6h second line
• Nifedipine: 10–20 mg daily–tid second line
• Amitriptyline: 10 mg PO tid second line
• Haloperidol: 2–10 mg IM second line

TABLE 12–19: Laceration

- Assess patient and check vitals

Immunization Status	Clean, Minor Wound		All Other Wounds	
	Tetanus-Diphtheria Toxoid (Td)	Tetanus Immuno-globulin (TIG)	Td	TIG
≥3 doses received in immunization series	Give only if last booster >10 yrs	No	If last booster >5 yrs	No*
<3 doses received or uncertain of immunization	Yes	No	Yes	Yes

- Td dosage: 0.5 mg IM × 1 dose
- Td and TIG should be given on two separate sites

*TIG is not given unless patient has humoral immune deficiency (e.g., HIV, agammaglobulinemia).
Source: From *MMWR Morb Mortal Wkly Rep* 1991;40(RR-10):1.

TABLE 12–20: N/V
• Phenergan: 12.5–25 mg IV/PO/IM/PR q4–6h *or*
• Prochlorperazine (Compazine): 5–10 mg IV over 2 mins, 5–10 mg PO/IM tid–qid, 25-mg suppository PR bid *or*
• Ondansetron (Zofran): 8 mg PO bid (if >12 yrs), 4 mg PO tid (if <12 yrs) *or*
• Trimethobenzamide (Tigan): 250 mg PO q6–8h, 200 mg IM/PR q6–8h *or*
• Reglan: 10 mg IV/IM q2–3h, 10–15 mg PO qid 30 mins before meal (recommended for patient with GI dysmotility)

TABLE 12–21: Pain Management

Note: Patient with DNR status → be liberal with pain medication when managing pain

Do not give Demerol with monoamine oxidase inhibitor (MAOI)— **it can kill a patient**

- Assess pain and document (location, intensity, quality, severity)

- Consider increasing pain medication dose if the patient is already on pain medication

- Search for etiology of pain → consider treating the cause of pain

- Be cautious of using opiates in patient with hypotension

Mild to moderate pain

- Tylenol: 325–650 mg PO/PR q4–6h (max: 4 g/24 hrs) *or*

- Codeine plus acetaminophen (30/300) (Tylenol #3): 1–2 tablets PO q4–6h *or*

- Tylenol with codeine elixir: 15 mL q4–6h *or*

- Salicylate

  ASA: 325–650 mg PO/PR q4–6h *or*

  Salsalate: 500–750 mg PO q8–12h *or*

- Propionic acids

  Ibuprofen: 200–600 mg PO q4–6h *or*

  Naproxen: 250–500 mg PO bid *or*

- Acetic acids

  Sulindac: 150–200 mg PO bid *or*

  Diclofenac: 50 mg PO bid–tid, 75 mg PO bid

Moderate pain

- Acetic acids: ketorolac (Toradol), 10 mg PO q4–6h, 15–30 mg IM/IV q6h (max: 5 days) *or*

- Opioid agonist:

  Codeine: 0.5–1.0 mg/kg (15–60 mg PO/IM/IV/SQ q4–6h PRN, oral solution, 15 mg/5 mL) *or*

(continued)

TABLE 12–21: Pain Management (Continued)
Propoxyphene: 65–100 mg PO q4h PRN *or*
• Opioid combination
Darvocet: 2 tablets PO q4h PRN *or*
Hydrocodone and acetaminophen (2.5/500) (Lortab): 1–2 tab PO q4–6h PRN *or*
Oxycodone and acetaminophen (2.5/325) (Percocet): 1–2 tab PO q6h PRN *or*
Oxycodone and ASA (5/325) (Percodan): 1 tab PO q6h PRN *or*
Hydrocodone and acetaminophen (5/500) (Vicodin): 1–2 tab PO q4–6h PRN
• Opioid agonist-antagonist
Pentazocine (Talwin): 30 mg IV/IM q3–4h PRN *or*
Pentazocine plus naloxone (50/0.5) (Talwin NX): 1 tablet PO q3–4h PRN *or*
Butorphanol (Stadol): 0.5–2.0 mg IV or 1–4 mg IM q3–4h PRN *or*
Stadol: 1 spray (1 mg) in 1 nostril q3–4h PRN
• Other
Tramadol (Ultram): 50–100 mg PO q4–6h PRN (seizure can occur with concurrent use of antidepressants and patient with history of seizure disorder)
Moderate to severe pain
• Morphine: 1–2 mg (max: 15 mg) IM/SQ or slow IV q4h PRN *or*
• Morphine CR (MS Contin): 30 mg PO q8–12h *or*
• Hydromorphone (Dilaudid): 2–4 mg PO q4–6h PRN *or*
0.5–2.0 mg IM/SQ or slow IV q4–6h PRN

(continued)

TABLE 12–21: Pain Management (Continued)

• Fentanyl [transdermal patch (Duragesic, Actiq)]: 25–100 mcg/hr (see Fentanyl Patch Dosing)

Note

• 1 mg Dilaudid = 7 mg morphine; 1 mg morphine = 7 mg Demerol

• If allergy to codeine → give Darvocet

• Darvocet is known to cause delirium in elderly

Pain Medications, Onset of Action, and Dosing Equivalents between PO and IV

Medication	Onset (mins)	Dosing (hrs)	Equivalents	
			Oral (mg)	IV (mg)
Codeine	10–30	4	200	120
Dilaudid	15–30	4	7.5	1.5
Levorphanol (Levo-Dromoran)	30–90	4	4	2
Demerol	10–45	4	300	75
Methadone	15–60	4	30	10
Morphine (Roxanol)	15–60	4	30	10
MS Contin	15–60	12	90	—
Oxycodone CR (OxyContin)	15–30	12	30	—
Propoxyphene	30–60	4	200	—

(continued)

TABLE 12–21: Pain Management (Continued)

Fentanyl Patch Dosing Compared to Other Narcotics, 1 mg = 1,000 mcg (Patch Takes 16 hrs to Take Effect)

Fentanyl	25 mcg/hr		50 mcg/hr		75 mcg/hr	
	PO/day	IM/day	PO/day	IM/day	PO/day	IV/day
Codeine (Tylenol plus codeine)	150–447	104–286	448–747	287–481	748–1,047	482–676
Oxycodone (Percocet)	22.5–67.0	12–33	67.5–112.0	33.1–56.0	112.5–157.0	56.1–78.0
Morphine	45–134	8–22	135–224	23–37	225–314	38–52
Dilaudid	5.6–17.0	1.2–3.4	17.1–28.0	3.5–5.6	28.1–39.0	5.7–7.9

Fentanyl	100 mcg/hr		125 mcg/hr		150 mcg/hr	
	PO/day	IV/day	PO/day	IV/day	PO/day	IM/day
Codeine (Tylenol plus codeine)	1,048–1,347	677–871	1,348–1,647	872–1,066	1,648–1,947	1,067–1,261
Oxycodone (Percocet)	157–202	78.1–101.0	202.5–247.0	101.1–123.0	247.5–292.0	123.1–147.0
Morphine	315–404	53–67	405–494	68–82	495–548	83–97
Dilaudid	39.1–51.0	8–10	51.1–62.0	10.1–12.0	62.1–73.0	12.1–15.0

TABLE 12–22: Sinus Pause
• Assess patient and check vitals
If <2.5 secs and asymptomatic → no treatment needed
If 2.5–3.0 secs and asymptomatic → atropine then epinephrine/ dopamine
External pacer at bedside
If >3 secs and asymptomatic → pacer placement required
If symptomatic → pacer placement required
• Atropine: 0.5–1.0 mg IV q3–5min (max: 0.04 mg/kg)
• Epinephrine: 2–10 mcg/min
• Dopamine: 5–20 mcg/kg/min

TABLE 12–23: Sleep Disturbance/Insomnia

- Restoril: 7.5 mg PO qhs *or*

- Zolpidem (Ambien): 5 mg PO qhs (good for patient requiring less sedation) *or*

- Trazodone (Desyrel): 50–100 mg PO qhs (use 25 mg in elderly) *or*

- Sonata: 10–20 mg PO qhs (half the dose in elderly and patient with liver disease) *or*

- Alprazolam (Xanax): 0.25 mg PO qhs (avoid in elderly or patient with delirium) *or*

- Benadryl: 25–50 mg PO qhs (avoid in elderly or patient with delirium)

TABLE 12–24: Tachycardia (>100)
• Assess patient and check vitals
• Check temperature (a high temperature can cause tachycardia)
• Ask for any symptoms: lightheadedness/dizziness/syncope/ palpitation/shortness of breath/chest pain
• Check ECG: check for arrhythmia; see Chapter 1 for management
• Review medications
• Manage appropriately
Note: Also see Table 1–9

TABLE 12–25: Unresponsive Patient
• Check code status
• ABCs
• Assess patient, check vitals, and O_2 saturation
• If BGM low (<55) → thiamine, 10 mg IV plus 1 amp of glucose $D_{50}W$ (1 amp can ↑ glucose by 100)
• Cardiac rhythm (12-lead ECG): look for arrhythmia, blocks, and MI
• CMP (chem 12) plus Mg
• ?Serum/urine toxicology
• If morphine-/other narcotic-induced → give Narcan, 0.2–2.0 mg IV/IM/SQ q5min
• If benzodiazepine-induced → give flumazenil, 0.2 mg IV over 30 secs
→ follow by 0.3 mg IV at 1 min → 0.5 mg IV at 2 mins
Note
• Flumazenil can cause seizure in patient who is on benzodiazepines chronically
• Flumazenil is contraindicated in hepatic encephalopathy
• Flumazenil may not be effective in chronic benzodiazepine users
• **Note:** Also see Table 11–1 and Table 12–6

Index

Page numbers followed by *f* indicate figures.